MW01680214

Statistical Tests in Medical Research

Jaykaran MD (Pharmacology), PGDRM
Assistant Professor
Department of Pharmacology
Government Medical College
Surat, Gujarat, India

Foreword

SK Vajpayee

JAYPEE BROTHERS MEDICAL PUBLISHERS (P) LTD

Ahmedabad • St Louis (USA) • Panama City (Panama) • London (UK) • New Delhi
Bengaluru • Chennai • Hyderabad • Kochi • Kolkata • Lucknow • Mumbai • Nagpur

Published by

Jitendar P Vij
Jaypee Brothers Medical Publishers (P) Ltd

Corporate Office
4838/24 Ansari Road, Daryaganj, **New Delhi** - 110002, India, Phone: +91-11-43574357
Fax: +91-11-43574314

Registered Office
B-3 EMCA House, 23/23B Ansari Road, Daryaganj, **New Delhi** - 110 002, India
Phones: +91-11-23272143, +91-11-23272703, +91-11-23282021
+91-11-23245672, Rel: +91-11-32558559, Fax: +91-11-23276490, +91-11-23245683
e-mail: jaypee@jaypeebrothers.com, Website: www.jaypeebrothers.com

Offices in India

- **Ahmedabad**, Phone: Rel: +91-79-32988717, e-mail: ahmedabad@jaypeebrothers.com
- **Bengaluru**, Phone: Rel: +91-80-32714073, e-mail: bangalore@jaypeebrothers.com
- **Chennai**, Phone: Rel: +91-44-32972089, e-mail: chennai@jaypeebrothers.com
- **Hyderabad**, Phone: Rel:+91-40-32940929, e-mail: hyderabad@jaypeebrothers.com
- **Kochi**, Phone: +91-484-2395740, e-mail: kochi@jaypeebrothers.com
- **Kolkata**, Phone: +91-33-22276415, e-mail: kolkata@jaypeebrothers.com
- **Lucknow**, Phone: +91-522-3040554, e-mail: lucknow@jaypeebrothers.com
- **Mumbai**, Phone: Rel: +91-22-32926896, e-mail: mumbai@jaypeebrothers.com
- **Nagpur**, Phone: Rel: +91-712-3245220, e-mail: nagpur@jaypeebrothers.com

Overseas Offices

- **North America Office, USA,** Ph: 001-636-6279734,
  e-mail: jaypee@jaypeebrothers.com, anjulav@jaypeebrothers.com
- **Central America Office, Panama City, Panama,** Ph: 001-507-317-0160,
  e-mail: cservice@jphmedical.com
  Website: www.jphmedical.com
- **Europe Office, UK,** Ph: +44 (0) 2031708910, e-mail: info@jpmedpub.com

Statistical Tests in Medical Research

© 2011, Jaypee Brothers Medical Publishers

All rights reserved. No part of this publication should be reproduced, stored in a retrieval system, or transmitted in any form or by any means: electronic, mechanical, photocopying, recording, or otherwise, without the prior written permission of the author and the publisher.

This book has been published in good faith that the material provided by author is original. Every effort is made to ensure accuracy of material, but the publisher, printer and author will not be held responsible for any inadvertent error (s). In case of any dispute, all legal matters are to be settled under Delhi jurisdiction only.

First Edition: **2011**

ISBN 978-93-5025-160-7

Typeset at JPBMP typesetting unit

Printed at Rajkamal Electric Press, Plot No. 2, Phase-IV, Kundli, Haryana.

Foreword

Medical research and statistics are very rightly considered inseparable as the research remains inconclusive unless it is authenticated by appropriate statistical analysis. Medical researchers often find themselves handicapped when it comes to apply statistical analysis of the data obtained in the research. But more serious omission encountered more frequently is their failure to plan to study before its commencement particularly its statistical aspects. This neglect is bound to lend them in a difficult situation of how to mange the data. There is umpteen number of books by highly experienced authors elaborating the intricacies of fundamental and applied statistics. Unfortunately, majority of the users are stuck-up in the beginning itself, as they are unable to pickup the most appropriate statistical test. The problem is confounded by the variety of parameters studied and more so due to existence of different variable.

The present compilation comes handy in the wake of above scenario. The author, a researcher himself, has meticulously and very precisely identified the most suitable statistical tests for all conceivable studies in the field of medical research. The presentation is aided with classical examples from various situations. I am convinced and confident that it will prove to be an essential guide to all researchers whether he/she is at a junior level or a more experienced one as well as from any of the area like experimental, clinical or epidemiological research. A word of caution is necessary for the prospective user to decide the applicable statistical producer while planning the study and not after its completion. Secondly, it is also advisable to refer to the procedure detail of each method from standard sources. I hope that from now on the task of the puzzled researchers will be made easy by availability of a much-needed friendly guide.

SK Vajpayee MD (Pharmacology)
Dean
Government Medical College
and New Civil Hospital
Surat, Gujarat, India

Preface

It is quite a difficult job for a medical researcher to apply an appropriate statistical test for his/her study. Moreover, the books regarding the subject "Biostatistics" have not explored the topic in detail and this make it an uphill task after referring these books. Nowadays, because of the availability of statistical software, statistical tests can be performed within the seconds but which test to choose for the analysis of data, is still a problem.

So, I am making an honest and humble effort to try to deal with this confusing and difficult job and make this comprehensible to the readers. All the steps which are needed in selection of statistical tests are explained in detail. Readers should read one chapter at a time and try to grasp the concept of that chapter with the help of exercise given in the book as well as looking at the examples given in different books of biostatistics.

I would like to acknowledge my parents, my wife and brother for supporting me in this task. I would also like to acknowledge Dr ND Kantharia, HOD, Department of Pharmacology, Government Medical College, Surat, Dr SD Mistry, Professor, Department of Pharmacology, Government Medical College, Jamnagar and all the staff members of Department of Pharmacology, Government Medical College, Surat for helping me in learning of basic concepts of statistics. I also extend my thanks to publishers of this book, M/s Jaypee Brothers Medical Publishers (P) Ltd, New Delhi, India, without their help and support the publication of this book could not have been possible.

Jaykaran

Contents

CHAPTER 1

Introduction

Dear friends,

Welcome to the world of biostatistics. I congratulate you for purchasing this book.

Statistics is considered as boring subject ("If I had only one day left to live, I would live it in my statistics class: it would seem so much longer"). General consensus is that statistics is difficult to understand ("have you heard about the statistics joke gone horribly wrong? Even the undergraduate could understand it").

I do believe that understanding of statistics is easy but it should be taught in different way. So this book has been written with the purpose of understanding the concepts of biostatistics.

In this book, we will learn the skill of selection of appropriate statistical tests. Various books related to the "how to use" of test of significance are available but very few of them are dealing with selection of appropriate test. Nowadays, various statistical softwares are also available but to use them we must know which test to choose for our data?

So most important thing for analysis of any data is to know which test of significance should be used. In this book we will try to explore this concept.

Selection of any test of significance involves three basic steps:

1. What kind of data we are dealing with?
2. Whether our data are following the normal distribution or not?
3. Selection of appropriate statistical test.

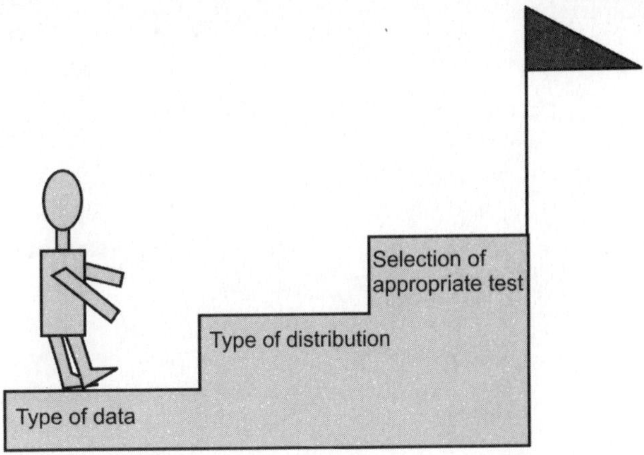

So, first of all it is necessary to understand the types of data.

CHAPTER 2

What Kind of Data We are Dealing with?

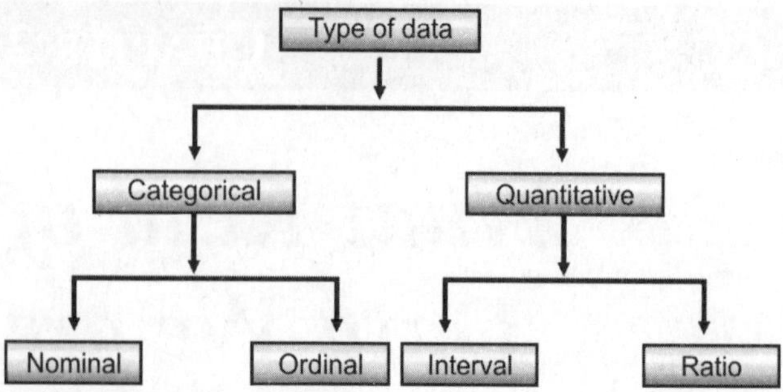

NOMINAL DATA

Data assigned with labels or names are considered as the data in nominal scale. Since, each label or name indicates a separate category in the data; this data is also called as categorical data. You can count but not order or measure nominal data. Nominal data are categorical data where the order of the categories is arbitrary. A good example is race/ethnicity has values 1 = White, 2 = Hispanic, 3 = American Indian, 4 = Black, 5 = other. Note that the order of the categories is arbitrary.

In the same way, we can calculate males and females in a class. Each individual will be either male or female. But there is no use of giving them rank order. When there are only two possible categories, the data is called dichotomous data like male/female, dead/alive, etc.

Examples of nominal data:

- Sex—male/female
- Alive/dead
- Blood groups—O, A, B, AB
- Prevented/not prevented
- Cured/not cured
- Infected/not infected

- Hair color—blonde, brown, red, black
- Race—Caucasian, African-American, Asian
- Smoking status—smoker, nonsmokers, etc

ORDINAL DATA

Ordinal data refers to data that has some meaningful order, so that, higher values represent more of some characteristic than lower values. For instance, in medical practice burns are commonly described by their degree, which describes the amount of tissue damage caused by the burn. A first-degree burn is characterized by redness of the skin, minor pain, and damage to the epidermis only, while a second-degree burn includes blistering and involves the dermis, and a third-degree burn is characterized by charring of the skin and possibly destroyed nerve endings. These categories may be ranked in a logical order: first-degree burns are the least serious in terms of tissue damage, third-degree burns the most serious. However, there is no metric analogous to a ruler or scale to quantify how great the distance between categories is, nor is it possible to determine if the difference between first- and second-degree burns is the same as the difference between second- and third-degree burn. Ordinal data are categorical data where there is a logical ordering to the categories. A good example is the Likert scale that you see on many surveys: 1 = Strongly disagree; 2 = Disagree; 3 = Neutral; 4 = Agree; 5 = Strongly agree.

Examples of ordinal data are:

- Various scales like—Hamilton depression scale, mini mental scale, etc.
- Grade of breast cancer
- Better, same, worse
- Disagree, neutral, agree

- Class—fresh, sophomore, junior, senior, supersenior
- Degree of illness—none, mild, moderate, severe
- Opinion of students about riots—ticked off, neutral, happy, etc.

INTERVAL DATA

Interval data has a meaningful order and also has the quality that equal intervals between measurements represent equal changes in the quantity of whatever is being measured. But these types of data have no natural zero. Example is celsius scale. In this particular scale, the unit of measurement is 1/100 of the difference between the melting temperature and the boiling temperature of water in atmospheric pressure. The "zero point" on an interval scale is arbitrary; and negative values can be used. IQ test is also interval data as it has no natural zero. People have different IQ level but nobody has IQ level of zero.

Natural Zero

Some scales of measurement have a natural zero and some do not. For example, height, weight, etc. have a natural 0 at no height or no weight. Consequently, it makes sense to say that 2 m is twice as large as 1m. Both of these variables are ratio scale. On the other hand, year and temperature (celsius) do not have a natural zero. The year 0 is arbitrary and it is not sensible to say that the year 2000 is twice as old as the year 1000. Similarly, 0°C is arbitrary and it again does not make sense to say that 20°C is twice as hot as 10°C. Both of these variables are interval scale.

RATIO DATA

Ratio data has all the qualities of interval data (natural order, equal intervals) plus a natural zero point. This is the most frequently used data. Physical measurements of height, weight, length are typically ratio variables. It is now meaningful to say that 10 m is twice as long as 5 m. This ratio hold true regardless of which scale the object is being measured in (e.g. meters or yards). This is because there is a natural zero. Another example is the Kelvin temperature scale which unlike celcius scale has a non-arbitrary zero point of absolute zero, which is denoted by °K and is equal to –273.15°C.

Examples are:

- Height
- Weight
- Length
- Blood pressure
- Blood cholesterol
- Hemoglobin level, etc.

To select the appropriate test you should able to differentiate nominal, ordinal and quantitative data.

Continuous and Discrete Data

Another distinction often made is that between continuous and discrete data. They are the subtype of quantitative data. Continuous data can take any value, or any value within a range. Most data measured by interval and ratio scales, other than that based on counting, is continuous: for instance, weight, height, distance, and income are all continuous. Discrete data can only take on particular values, and has clear boundaries. You can have 2 children or 3 children, but not 2.37 children, so "number of children" is a discrete variable.

Conversion of One Type of Data to Another

Quantitative data can be converted to categorical data by using "cut off points". For example, blood pressure can be turned into a nominal variable by defining "hypertension" as a diastolic blood pressure greater than 90 mm Hg, and "normotension" as blood pressure less than or equal to 90 mm Hg. Height (continuous) can be converted into "short", "average" or "tall" (ordinal). In general it is easier to summarize categorical variables, and so quantitative variables are often converted to categorical ones for descriptive purposes. To make a clinical decision on someone, one does not need to know the exact serum sodium level (continuous) but whether it is within the normal range (nominal). It may be easier to think of the proportion of the population who are hypertensive than the distribution of blood pressure. However, categorizing a continuous variable reduces the amount of information available and statistical tests will in general be more sensitive for a continuous variable than the corresponding nominal one, although more assumptions may have to be made about the data. Categorizing data is, therefore useful, for summarizing results, but not for statistical analysis.

Summarization of the types of the data:

Property	*Nominal data*	*Ordinal data*	*Interval data*	*Ratio data*
Logical order		Yes	Yes	Yes
Meaningful group interval			Yes	Yes
Meaningful ratio				Yes
True zero				Yes

Summarization of various statistical functions which can be calculated from data:

Ok to compute	*Nominal*	*Ordinal*	*Interval*	*Ratio*
Frequency distribution	Yes	Yes	Yes	Yes
Median and Percentiles	No	Yes	Yes	Yes
Add or Subtract	No	No	Yes	Yes
Mean, Standard deviation, Standard error of the mean	No	No	Yes	Yes
Ratio, or Coefficient of variation	No	No	Yes	Yes

EXERCISE

Fill in the blanks:

1. Data which has natural order, equal interval and natural zero is ....
2. Data in which each label or name indicate separate category is ....
3. Data which has natural order, equal interval but not natural zero is ....
4. Data which has meaningful order is ....
5. Data which can be counted but cannot be placed in meaningful order is ....
6. Celsius scale is .... type of data.
7. Nominal and ordinal are the .... type of data.
8. Interval and ratio are the .... type of data.
9. Hamilton depression scale, Likert scale and mini mental scales are .... types of data.
10. Categorizing of quantitative data is useful for ...., but not for statistical analysis.
11. Blood pressure is .... type of data.
12. "Normotensive"/"Hypertensive" are .... type of data.
13. Normal blood pressure/mildly raized blood pressure/moderately raized blood pressure are .... type of data.
14. .... of statistical test is more with continuous data as compared to categorical data.
15. "Continuous" and "discrete" are subtype of .... data.
16. Data which can only take on particular values, and has clear boundaries are .... data.
17. Data which can take any value, or any value within a range are .... data.

Answers

1. Ratio data
2. Nominal data
3. Interval data
4. Ordinal data
5. Nominal data
6. Interval
7. Categorical
8. Quantitative
9. Ordinal
10. Summarizing results
11. Ratio
12. Nominal
13. Ordinal
14. Sensitivity
15. Quantitative
16. Discrete
17. Continuous

Identify the type of data:
(A-Nominal, B-Ordinal, C-Interval, D-Ratio)

1. Grade of breast cancer ________
2. Weight ________
3. Cured/not cured ________
4. Degree of illness—none, mild, moderate, severe ________
5. Blood cholesterol ________
6. Sex—male/female ________
7. Height ________
8. Better, same, worse ________
9. Disagree, neutral, agree ________
10. Smoking status—smoker, nonsmokers ________
11. Blood pressure ________
12. Opinion of students about riots—ticked off, neutral, happy ________
13. Hemoglobin level ________
14. Alive/dead ________
15. Blood groups—O, A, B, AB ________
16. Prevented/not prevented ________
17. Length ________
18. Infected/not infected, etc. ________

19. Hair color—blonde, brown, red, black ________
20. Race— Caucasian. African-American, Asian _____
21. Class—fresh, sophomore, junior, senior, super senior ________
22. Celsius scale of temperature ________
23. Kelvin scale of temperature ________

Answers

1. B	2. D	3. A	4. B	5. D	6. A
7. D	8. B	9. B	10. A	11. D	12. B
13. D	14. A	15. A	16. A	17. D	18. A
19. A	20. A	21. B	22. C	23. D	

True/False exercise (tick the correct one):

1. Continuous and discrete are the subtype of categorical data. *True/False*
2. In ordinal data the rank order is always meaningful. *True/False*
3. Continuous data should be converted into the categorical data to analyze them. *True/False*
4. We can count the nominal data but cannot give them meaningful order. *True/False*
5. The only difference between interval data and ratio data is natural zero. *True/False*
6. For summarizing the results, quantitative data can be converted into the categorical one. *True/False*
7. Continuous data are the data which can have only particular value, cannot have the fractions. *True/False*
8. Ordinal data have equal interval between two rank orders. *True/False*
9. Interval and ratio data have equal interval between two values. *True/False*

10. Celsius scale of temperature is ordinal data.
True/False

Answers

1. False	2. True	3. False	4. True
5. True	6. True	7. False	8. False
9. True	10. False		

Identify the Type of Data from Statistical Problems

During analysis of results from any research, first thing we must know is type of data. So, now some problems are explained below. You are supposed to identify only the type of data as this is the first stage of selection of appropriate statistical test-

1. Ten individuals are chosen at random from a normal population and there weights in kg are found to be—70, 56, 65, 49, 79, 56, 80, 58, 69 and 73. Does this sample adequately represent a population in which the mean weight was found to be—70 kg?

Type of data: ....

2. From the data given in table, test whether the prevalence of scabies, in two different sexes is significantly different.

Sex	*No. with scabies*	*No. without scabies*	*Total*
Male	1168	10200	11368
Female	600	7900	8500
Total	1768	18100	19868

Type of data: ....

3. In a clinical trial to assess the efficacy of new antianxiety drugs on patients of anxiety disorders with each patient being given a week's treatment with drug. The drug was considered effective if, it lowered anxiety score after treatment. Test the efficacy of drug on the following results.

Before treatment—22, 18, 17, 19, 22, 12, 10, 11, 19, 8

After treatment—19, 20, 11, 9, 22, 15, 20, 20, 6, 7

Type of data: ....

4. Chest circumference in centimeters of 12 normal children and 12 malnourished children aged one year are given

below. Test for the statistical significance of the difference in chest circumference, on an average between these two groups.

Normal groups—43, 47, 50, 52, 34, 48, 51, 43, 50, 39, 47, 44

Malnourished group—38, 41, 36, 35, 30, 42, 31, 29, 31, 35, 40, 36

Type of data: ....

5. During a nutrition survey in a random sample of 1000 people, nutritional status found to be as below:

Excellent	160
Good	200
Fair	270
Poor	370
Total	1000

Type of data: ....

6. Does any sex partner play any role for the positivity of HIV?

Sex partner	*HIV*		
	+ve	*–ve*	*Total*
Male	0	8	8
Female	13	311	324
Both	1	6	7
Total	14	325	339

Type of data: ....

7. During a laboratory experiment muscular contractions of a frog muscle were measured against different doses of a given drug. The height of curve was considered as the response to the drug. The observations were as below:

	Serial no. of experiments				
	1	2	3	4	5
Dose of drug	0.3	0.4	0.6	0.8	0.9
Response to drug	54.0	59.0	60.0	65.0	70.0

Type of data: ....

8. A group of 20 normal children in a study had a mean serum iron level of 148 microgram percentage and SD of 44.03. Another group of 20 children with infantile cirrhosis of liver had mean serum iron level of 150 microgram percentages and SD of 49.04%. Is the difference between the two means statistically significant?

Type of data: ....

9. Thirty-five microgram of vitamin B_{12} were given intramuscularly every fourth to sixth week patients of pernicious anemia during period of remission. The results are given below. Do the data indicate real improvement in hemoglobin level?

Individual number	*Hemoglobin gm%*	
	Before therapy	*After 3 months of therapy*
1	12.2	13.0
2	11.3	13.4
3	14.7	16.0
4	11.4	13.6
5	11.5	14.0
6	12.7	13.8

Type of data: ....

10. From a population 50 females using oral contraceptives and 60 female using other contraceptives devices were randomly selected and number of hypertensive cases from

both the were recorded as given below. Test the hypothesis that proportion of patients with hypertension is the same for two groups.

Type of contraceptive	*Total*	*No. found hypertensive*
Oral	50	8
Other	60	16

Type of data: ....

Answers

1. Ratio
2. Nominal
3. Ordinal
4. Ratio
5. Ordinal
6. Nominal
7. Ratio
8. Ratio
9. Ratio
10. Nominal

Dear readers, by now you must have got a fair idea about the identification of types of data. If you feel that your concepts are not up to the mark and you are facing problem in identification of data than donot proceed further. Read the theory part again and again. You can take the help of some statistician, but don't proceed to next chapter without understanding these concepts. If you are good in identification of data, you are half way to your goal of selection of appropriate test.

As you know, understanding the use of appropriate statistical test serve two purposes. One, to acquire skill for analysis of data in our research and second, to interpret the quality of paper published in journals. The papers published in various journals are full of statistical flaws and a good knowledge of statistics is necessary to understand the validity of results. After the completion of this book you will able to analyze the articles published in journals for there appropriateness of statistical tests.

So now we will try to understand and identify type of data which are published in some peer reviewed journals. Remember the first step for appropriateness of statistical test is identification of type of data, later we will talk about the selection of tests.

1. Effect of Fresh *Triticum Aestivum* Grass Juice on Lipid Profile of Normal Rats

Objective: To study the hypolipidemic activity of fresh grass juice of Triticum aestivum in normal rats.

Materials and methods: Freshly prepared *Triticum aestivum* grass juice was administered to normal rats at the dose of 5 ml/kg and 10 ml/kg orally once daily for 21 days. Blood samples were collected after 24 hours of last administration and used for estimation of lipid profile (TC: Total cholesterol, TG: Triglyceride, HDL: High density lipoprotein, LDL: Low density lipoprotein, VLDL: Very low density lipoprotein).

So, here researchers wants to see the effect of grass juice on lipid parameters. Can you identify the type of data? (nominal or ordinal or interval or ratio).

Type of data in this study is ....

(Kothari S, Jain AK, Mehta SC, Tonpay SD. Effect of Fresh *Triticum Aestivum* Grass Juice on Lipid Profile of Normal Rats. Indian J Pharmacol 2008;40:235-6).

2. Verbal and Visual Memory in Patients with Early Parkinson's Disease: Effect of Levodopa

Background: The effect of initiation of levodopa therapy on the memory functions in patients with Parkinson's disease remains poorly understood.

Aims: To evaluate the effect of initiation of levodopa therapy on memory, in patients with early Parkinson's disease.

Settings and Design: Prospective case control study.

Materials and methods: Seventeen patients with early Parkinson's disease were evaluated for verbal memory using Rey's auditory verbal learning test, and visual memory using the Benton's visual retention test and form sequence learning test. UPDRS scores, Hoehn and Yahr's Staging and Schwab and England scores of activities of daily living. Hamilton's depression rating scale and MMSE were also evaluated. Six controls were also evaluated according to similar study protocol. Levodopa was then prescribed to the cases. Same tests were repeated on all the subjects after 12 weeks.

In this study researcher saw the effect of levodopa on various scores like UPDRS, MMSE (mini mental scale), HDRS (Hamilton depression scale). So, you have to find which type of data scales are.

Type of data in this study is ....

(Singh S, Behari M. Verbal and Visual Memory in Patients with early Parkinson's Disease: Effect of Levodopa. Neurol India 2006;54:33-7).

3. Evaluation of the Analgesic Effect of Salmon Calcitonin in Metastatic Bone Pain

Aim: To evaluate the efficacy of calcitonin in controlling metastatic bone pain.

Materials and methods: Patients with bone metastases, with a numerical pain score greater than 4 were randomized to receive calcitonin 200 IU subcutaneously 6 hourly for 48 hours (n = 10) or normal saline placebo (n = 10). The parameter measured were the 11-point numerical pain score by a blinded investigator.

Type of data: ....

(Mishra S, Bhatnagar S, Jha RR. Evaluation of the Analgesic Effect of Salmon Calcitonin in Metastatic Bone Pain. Indian J Palliat Care 2003;9:8-13).

4. Adverse Drug Reaction Profile of Different Antiretroviral Agents

Background: The introduction of highly active antiretroviral therapy (HAART) has led to significant reduction in acquired immune deficiency syndrome (AIDS) related morbidity and mortality. Adverse drug reactions (ADRs) to antiretroviral treatment (ART) are however, major obstacles in its success.

Aims: Authors sought to study the adverse effects of ART in a resource restricted setting in India.

Methods: Hundred patients on ART were studied prospectively over a period of two years. All patients were asked to visit the clinic if they developed any symptoms or on a monthly basis. They were screened clinically and investigated suitably for any ADRs.

Result table:

Drug (No. of cases)	*Cases with ADR (%)*
AZT (42)	21 (50)
d4T (48)	23 (47.9)
3TC (90)	01 (1.1)
NVP (76)	14 (18.4)
EFV (11)	05 (45.4)

Type of data in this study is ....

(Marfatia Y.S, Makrandi S. Adverse Drug Reactions Due to Antiretrovirals: Issues and Challenges. Indian J Sex Transm Dis 2005; 26:1-2)

5. Comparison of Weight-Loss Diets with Different Compositions of Fat, Protein, and Carbohydrates

Background: The possible advantage for weight loss of a diet that emphasizes protein, fat, or carbohydrates has not been established, and there are few studies that extend beyond 1 year.

Methods: Researchers randomly assigned 811 overweight adults to one of four diets; the targeted percentages of energy derived from fat, protein, and carbohydrates in the four diets were 20, 15, and 65%; 20, 25, and 55%; 40, 15, and 45%; and 40, 25, and 35%. The diets consisted of similar foods and met guidelines for cardiovascular health. The participants were offered group and individual instructional sessions for 2 years. The primary outcome was the change in body weight after 2 years in two-by-two factorial comparisons of low fat versus high fat and average protein versus high protein and in the comparison of highest and lowest carbohydrate content.

Type of data in this study is ....

(Sacks FM, et al. Comparison of Weight-Loss Diets with Different Compositions of Fat, Protein, and Carbohydrates N. Engl J Med, February 26,2009;360(9):859-73).

6. Current and Former Marijuana Use: Preliminary Findings of a Longitudinal Study of Effects on IQ in Young Adults

Background: Assessing marijuana's impact on intelligence quotient (IQ) has been hampered by a lack of evaluation of subjects before they begin to use this substance. Using data from a group of young people whom authors have been following since birth, authors examined IQ scores before, during and after cessation of regular marijuana use to determine any impact of the drug on this measure of cognitive function.

Methods: Authors determined marijuana use for seventy, 17 to 20-year-olds through self-reporting and urinalysis. IQ difference scores were calculated by subtracting each person's IQ score at 9 to12 years (before initiation of drug use) from his or her score at 17 to 20 years. Researchers then compared the difference in IQ scores of current heavy users (at least 5 joints per week), current light users (less than 5 joints per week), former users (who had not smoked regularly for at least 3 months) and non-users (who never smoked more than once per week and no smoking in the past two weeks).

So, what kind of data IQ is?

Type of data in this study is ....

(Fried P, et al. Current and Former Marijuana use: Preliminary Findings of a Longitudinal Study of Effects on IQ in Young Adults. Cmaj 2002;166(7):887-91).

7. Drug-Eluting Stents Vs Coronary Artery Bypass Grafting in Multivessel Coronary Disease

Background: Numerous studies have compared the outcomes of two competing interventions for multivessel coronary artery disease: Coronary artery bypass grafting (CABG) and coronary stenting. However, little information has become available since the introduction of drug-eluting stents.

Methods: Authors identified patients with multivessel disease who received drug-eluting stents or underwent CABG in New York State between October 1st, 2003, and December 31st, 2004, and they compared adverse outcomes (death or myocardial infarction, or repeat avoid loose revascularization) through December 31st, 2005, after adjustment for differences in baseline risk factors among the patients.

Type of data in this study is ....

(Hannan EL, Wu C, Walford G, Culliford AT, Gold JP, Smith CR, et al. Drug-Eluting Stents vs Coronary Artery Bypass Grafting in Multivessel Coronary Disease. N Engl J Med 2008;358:331-41).

8. Effect of Shilajit on Blood Glucose and Lipid Profile in Alloxan-induced Diabetic Rats

Objective: To study the effect of shilajit (a herbomineral preparation) on blood glucose and lipid profile in euglycemic and alloxan-induced diabetic rats and its effects on the above parameters in combination with conventional antidiabetic drugs.

Material and methods: Diabetes was induced in albino rats by administration of a single dose of alloxan monohydrate 5% (125 mg/kg, i.p.). Effects of three different doses of shilajit (50, 100 and 200 mg/kg/day, orally), alone for 4 weeks and a combination of shilajit (100 mg/kg/day, orally) with either glibenclamide (5 mg/kg/day, orally) or metformin (0.5 g/kg/day, orally) for 4 weeks were studied on blood glucose and lipid profile.

Type of data in this study is ....

(Trivedi NA, Mazumdar B, Bhatt JD, Hemavathi KG. Effect of Shilajit on Blood Glucose and Lipid Profile in Alloxan-induced Diabetic Rats. Indian J Pharmacol 2004;36:373-6).

9. Aprotinin during Coronary Artery Bypass Grafting and Risk of Death

Background: Aprotinin (Trasylol) is used to mitigate bleeding during coronary artery bypass grafting (CABG). Accumulating evidence suggests that this practice increases mortality.

Methods: Using electronic administrative records of the premier perspective comparative database, authors studied hospitalized patients with operating room charges for the use of aprotinin (33,517 patients) or aminocaproic acid (44,682 patients) on the day CABG was performed. They tabulated the numbers of patients with a hospital discharge status of death and performed three types of analyses: A multivariable logistic regression analysis (primary analysis); propensity score matching in the highly selected subcohort of patients who received full amounts of the study drug, who underwent CABG by surgeons who performed 50 or more CABG surgeries during the study period, and for whom information on 10 additional covariates was available because the surgery occurred on hospital day 3 or later; and an instrumental-variable analysis of data from patients whose surgeons showed a strong preference for one of the two study drugs.

Type of data in this study is ....

(Schneeweiss S, Seeger JD, Landon J. Aprotinin During Coronary Artery Bypass Grafting and Risk of Death. NEJM 2008;358:771-83).

10. Is Combination Olanzapine and Antidepressant Medication Associated with a More Rapid Response Trajectory than Antidepressant Alone?

Objective: The authors' goal was to determine if prescription of antidepressant medication plus olanzapine initiates a more rapid response than prescription of antidepressant alone.

Method: Twenty patients with major depression were studied. For 2 weeks the patients were blindly assigned to receive antidepressant plus olanzapine or antidepressant plus placebo. After 2 weeks, olanzapine augmentation was initiated for patients who did not improve with placebo augmentation. Response to medication was measured primarily by Hamilton depression rating scale score.

Results:

Depression variable	*Placebo (N-10)*	*Olanzapine (N-10)*
Baseline Hamilton depression rating scale	23.6 ± 5.7	20.5 ± 4.6
Day 7: Hamilton depression rating scale	13.6 ± 6.5	11.3 ± 6.1
Day 14: Hamilton depression rating scale	13.5 ± 7.2	8.4 ± 3.6

Type of data in this study is ....

(Parker G, Brotchie H, Parker K. Is Combination Olanzapine and Antidepressant Medication Associated with a More Rapid Response Trajectory than Antidepressant Alone? Am J Psychiatry 2005;162:796-98).

11. Effect of Fluoxetine on Some Cognitive Functions of Patients of Depression

Background: This study was carried out to evaluate the effect of long term administration of a commonly prescribed antidepressants, fluoxetine on memory and psychomotor functions in patients of various psychiatric disorders using a battery of simple tests that can be conveniently applied to the Indian population.

Methods: Memory was evaluated using the P.G.I. memory scale and psychomotor functions were evaluated using six letter cancellation test (SLCT). Memory functions were evaluated at baseline, after 15 days and after 1 month.

Type of data in this study is ....

(Jaykaran, Bhardwaj P, Kantharia ND, Yadav P, Panwar A. Effect of Fluoxetine on Some Cognitive Functions of Patients of Depression. Indian J Psychol Med;2009,31:24-9).

Answers

1. Ratio
2. Ordinal
3. Ordinal
4. Nominal
5. Ratio
6. Interval
7. Nominal
8. Ratio
9. Nominal
10. Ordinal
11. Ordinal

CHAPTER 3

Whether Our Data are Following the Normal Distribution or Not?

This is the second prerequisite for selection of appropriate statistical test. If you know the type of data (nominal, ordinal, interval and ratio) and distribution of data (normal distribution or not normal distribution) than selection of statistical test will be very easy.

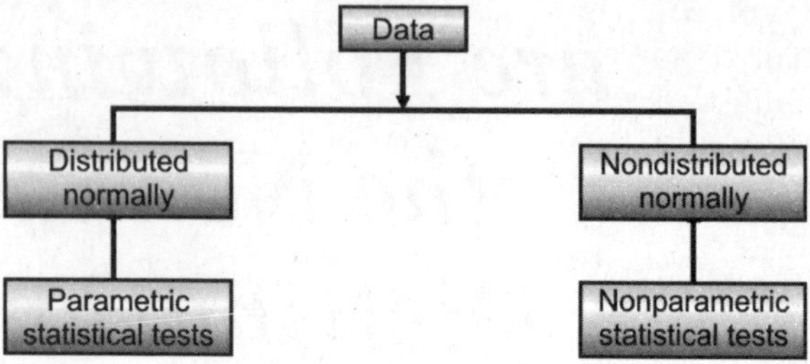

So, the simplified approach is—if your data are following the normal distribution then parametric statistical test should be used and nonparametric tests should be used when normal distribution is not followed.

There are various types of statistical tests used for the analysis of data following the normal distribution (parametric tests). Each parametric test has an equivalent nonparametric test which is used in the analysis of data not following the normal distribution is as follows:

Parametric tests	Equivalent nonparametric tests
One-sample *t* test	Wilcoxon test
Unpaired *t* test	Mann-Whitney test
Paired *t* test	Wilcoxon test
One-way ANOVA	Kruskal-Wallis test
Repeated-measures ANOVA	Friedman test

(Contd.)

(*Contd.*)

Pearson correlation	Spearman correlation
Simple linear regression or Nonlinear regression	Nonparametric regression

We will understand these tests further in next section. Here you just remember that if data are distributed normally than parametric tests should be used and if not distributed normally than nonparametric tests should be used. For example, if your data is not distributed normally than at the place of unpaired *t* test you will use Mann-Whitney test (see table).

Now, the question is how to check the data for normal distribution?

CHECKING THE DATA FOR NORMAL DISTRIBUTION

It is very important for us to understand that not all types of data should be checked for normal distribution.

Nominal data: There is no need to check for normal distribution in nominal data as it is very clear that they follow the chi-square distribution.

Ordinal data: There is no need to check distribution for ordinal data as these kinds of data contains rank or order and they do not follow the normal distribution.

> So, distribution of data should be checked only in the case of interval and ratio data.

There are various methods for checking the normal distribution. Some of methods are too complex to explain here. So, here we will use the simplified approach. Distribution of data can be checked by:

1. By measuring skewness and kurtosis
2. By plotting the histogram
3. By using statistical tests like: Komolgorov Smirnov test *and* Shapiro Wilk test.

1. Measuring Skewness and Kurtosis

I hope you must be aware of the characteristics of a normal distribution curve (read the standard book of biostatistics if you do not know).

Skewness

This is how a normal distribution curve looks like as in Figure 3.1.

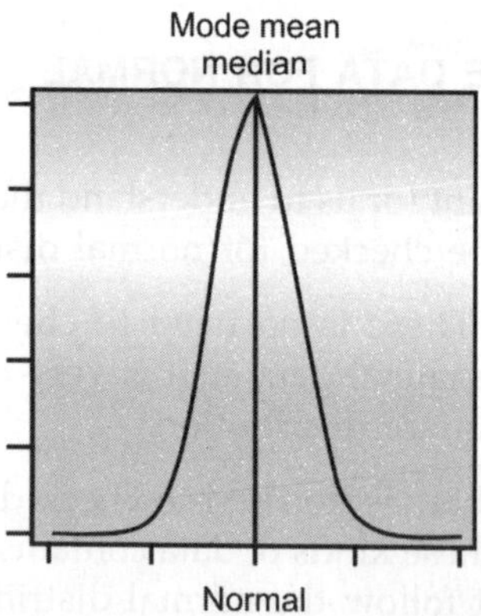

Fig. 3.1: Normal distribution curve. You can see mean, median and mode coincide at same point

Sometime data do not follow the normal distribution and upper curve shifted to left or right. That is called skewness as shown in Figures 3.2 and 3.3.

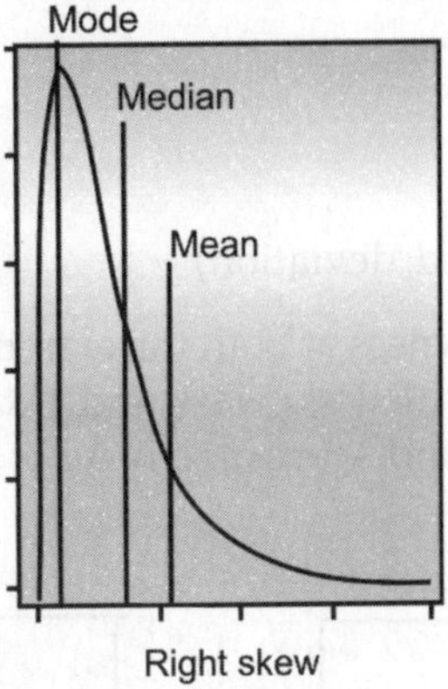

Fig. 3.2: This is right side skewness. See the position of mean, median and mode

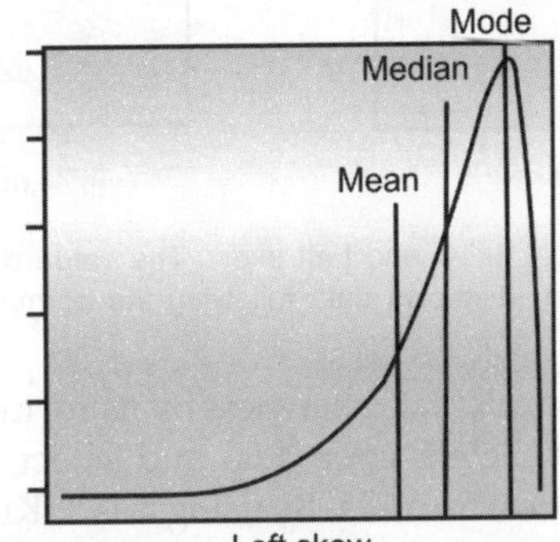

Fig. 3.3: This is left side skewness. Mean, median and mode shifted to opposite as compared to right side skewness

The formula for calculation of skewness is:

$$\frac{\Sigma (X-\mu)^3}{N\sigma^3}$$

μ: Mean
σ: SD (standard deviation)

The value of skewness at both the extreme conditions like extremely right sided skewess and extremely left sided skewness is +3 and –3 respectively is shown below in Figure 3.4.

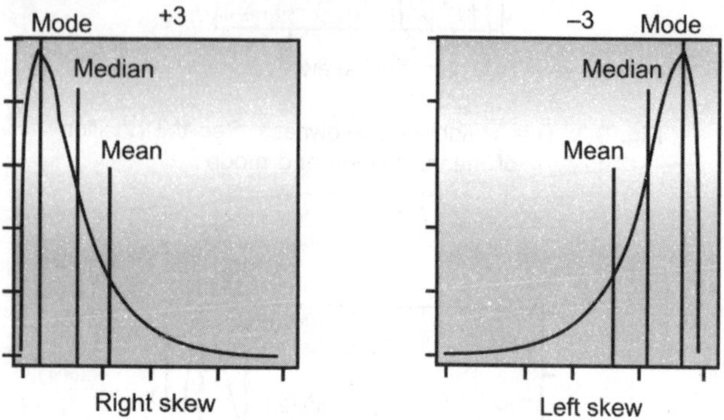

Fig. 3.4: Right skew and Left skew. The value of skewness between +1 to –1 shows data following the normal distribution

You can also calculate skewness by using microsoft excel function sheet. Select your data and select the "SKEW" from the statistical formula. By using this "SKEW" function you can get exact value of skewness. If this value is between +1 to –1, than your data are following the normal distribution. But other test of normality should also be performed to validate this. Skewness can also calculated with the help of any statistical software.

Kurtosis (Peakedness)

Degree of peakedness relative to the length and size of tails is kurtosis as shown in Figure 3.5

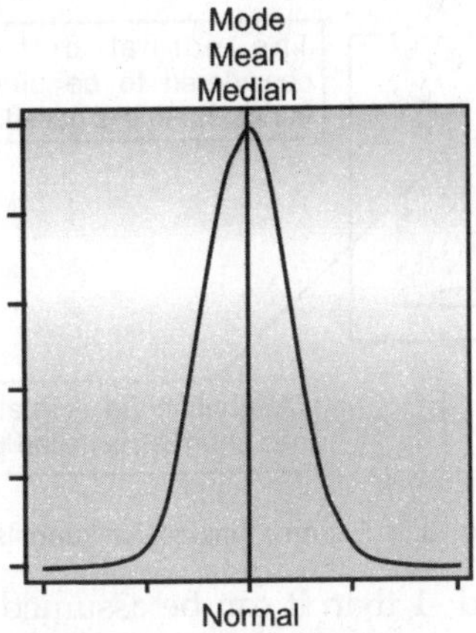

Fig. 3.5: Normal distribution curve

The formula for calculation of kurtosis is:

$$\frac{\Sigma (X-\mu)^4}{N\sigma^4} - 3$$

μ: Mean

σ: SD (standard deviation)

As you can see in Figure 3.6 the extreme value for kurtosis is +3 to –3. +3 for the highest peak and –3 for lowest.

> The value of kurtosis between +1 to –1 show the data are following the normal distribution.

Like skewness, kurtosis can also be calculated from microsoft excel sheet. You should select "KURT" function from the statistical functions given there. If value is in

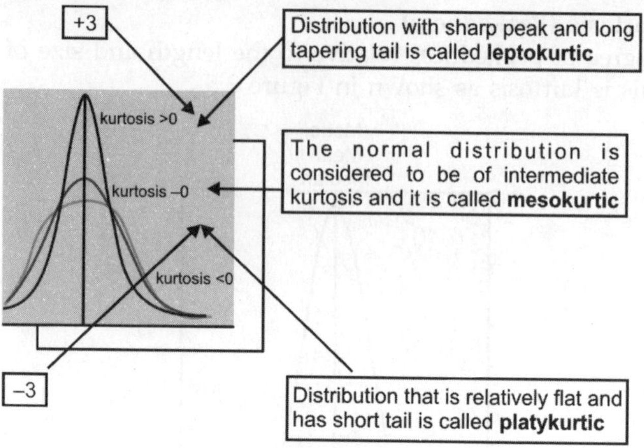

Fig. 3.6: Extreme values for kurtosis

between +1 and -1 than it can be assumed that data are following the normal distribution. Again it should be confirmed by other tests of normality. Kurtosis can also be calculated from the statistical software.

2. By Plotting the Histogram

Idea about the normal distribution can be generated by looking at the histogram (read the standard books for method of plotting the histogram). But this generates a rough idea and decision about the normal distribution should not be taken just on the basis of histogram (Figs 3.7 to 3.10).

3. By Using Statistical Tests like Kolmogorov-Smirnov Test and Shapiro-Wilk Test

There are various other tests available but these are most frequently used tests for checking the distribution of data. How to use these tests are beyond the scope of this book

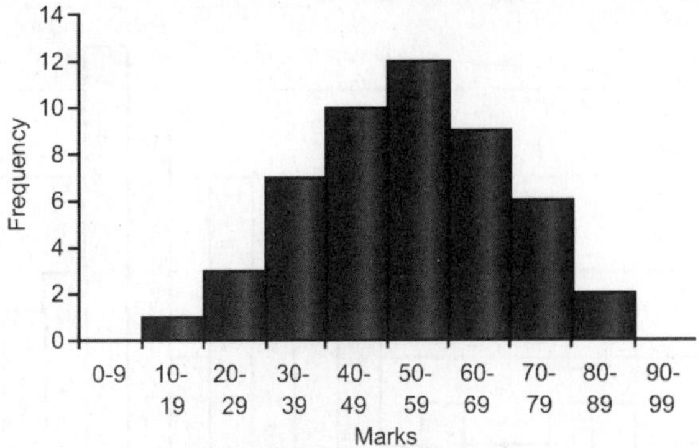

Fig. 3.7: Frequency histogram

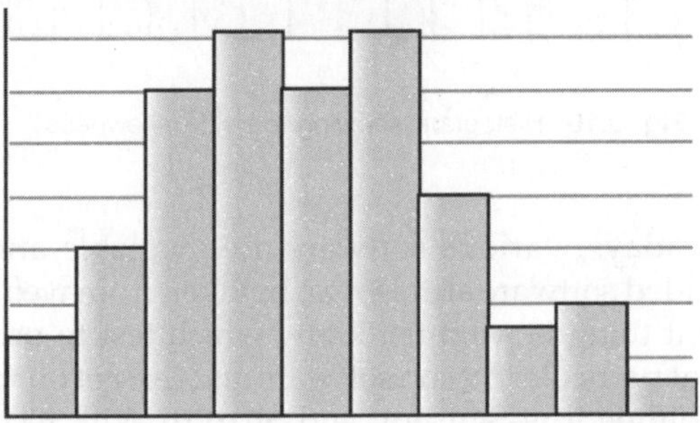

Fig. 3.8: Histogram showing the normal distribution

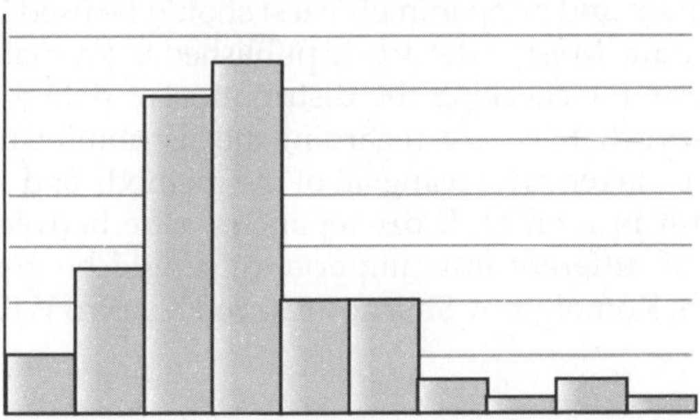

Fig. 3.9: Histogram showing right side skewness

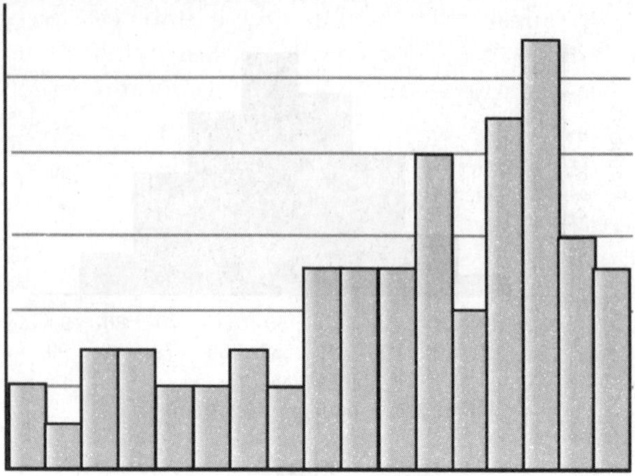

Fig. 3.10: Histogram showing left side skewness

but nowadays, various software are available and free downloaded software are also can be taken from web. Most important thing is we must know which test to use, and select that particular test on software and can get our result.

In, Kolmogorov-Smirnov and Shapiro-Wilk test if, P-value is less than 0.05 then data is not following the normal distribution and nonparametric test should be used in that kind of data. Most of the article published in journals uses these tests for checking the distribution of data.

I believe that decision regarding the distribution of data should be taken after using all of the methods and seeing the result in totality. If discrepancies arise between the results of different tests importance should be given to results of Komolgorov Smirnov test and Shapiro Wilk test.

As we already discussed that there is no need to check distribution in nominal and ordinal data as nominal follows the Chi-square distribution and ordinal data are considered of not following the normal distributions. Distribution should be checked in interval and ordinal data.

Checking Distribution of Data: A Simplified Approach

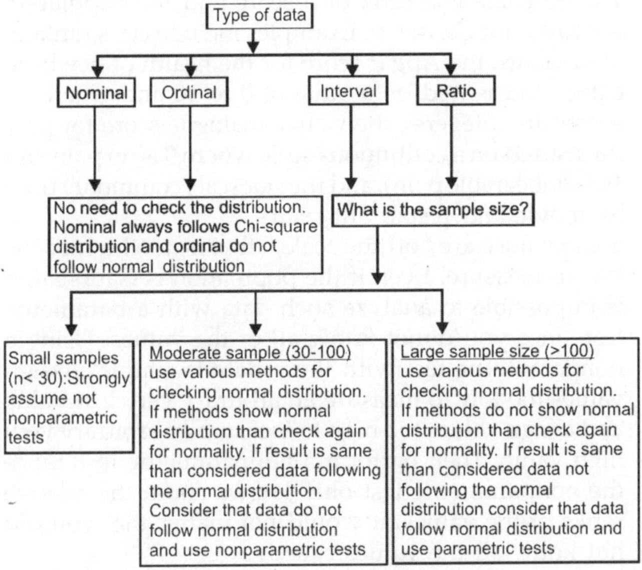

*Sample size is very important for analyzing the distribution of data. Less size (< 30) almost always does not follow the normal distribution. Moderate sample size (30-100) usually does not follow the normal distribution that's why data should be analyzed again for distribution if initial test results indicate normal distribution. In the case of large sample size (> 100) usually data are distributed normally. So, if normality tests show non, normal distribution then they should be analyzed again. Sometime data are converted by using log scale or reciprocal from non-normal to normal.

CHOOSING BETWEEN PARAMETRIC AND NONPARAMETRIC TESTS: THE EASY CASES

Choosing between parametric and nonparametric tests is sometimes easy. You should definitely choose a parametric test if you are sure that your data are sampled from a population that follows a Gaussian distribution, (at least approximately). You should definitely select a nonparametric test in three situations:

1. The outcome is a rank or a score and the population is clearly not Gaussian. Examples include class ranking of students, the Apgar score for the health of newborn babies (measured on a scale of 0 to 10 and where all scores are integers), the visual analogue score for pain (measured on a continuous scale where 0 is no pain and 10 is unbearable pain), and the star scale commonly used by movie and restaurant critics.
2. Some values are "off the scale," that is, too high or too low to measure. Even if the population is Gaussian, it is impossible to analyze such data with a parametric test since you donot know all of the values. Using a nonparametric test with these data is simple. Assign values too low to measure an arbitrary very low value and assign values too high to measure an arbitrary very high value. Then perform a nonparametric test. Since the nonparametric test only knows about the relative ranks of the values, it would not matter that you did not know all the values exactly.
3. You are sure that the population is not distributed in a Gaussian manner. If the data are not sampled from a Gaussian distribution, consider whether you can transformed the values to make the distribution become Gaussian. For example, you might take the logarithm or reciprocal of all values. There are often biological or chemical reasons (as well as statistical ones) for performing a particular transform.

CHOOSING BETWEEN PARAMETRIC AND NONPARAMETRIC TESTS: THE HARD CASES

It is not always easy to decide whether a sample comes from a Gaussian population. Consider these points:

1. If you collect many data points (over a hundred or so), you can look at the distribution of data and it will be fairly obvious whether the distribution is approximately bell-shaped. A formal statistical test (Kolmogorov-Smirnoff test) can be used to test whether the distribution of the data differs significantly from a Gaussian distribution. With few data points, it is difficult to tell whether the data are Gaussian by inspection, and the formal test has little power to discriminate between Gaussian and non-Gaussian distributions.
2. You should look at previous data as well. Remember, what matters is the distribution of the overall population, not the distribution of your sample. In deciding whether a population is Gaussian, look at all available data, not just data in the current experiment.
3. Consider the source of scatter. When the scatter comes from the sum of numerous sources (with no one source contributing most of the scatter), you expect to find a roughly Gaussian distribution. When in doubt, some people choose a parametric test (because they are not sure the Gaussian assumption is violated), and others choose a nonparametric test (because they are not sure the Gaussian assumption is met).

CHOOSING BETWEEN PARAMETRIC AND NONPARAMETRIC TESTS: DOES IT MATTER?

Does it matter whether you choose a parametric or nonparametric test? The answer depends on sample size. There are four cases to think about:

1. Large sample: What happens when you use a parametric test with data from a non-Gaussian population? The central limit theorem ensures that parametric tests work well with large samples even if the population is non-Gaussian. In other words, parametric tests are robust to deviations from Gaussian distributions, so long as the samples are large. The snag is that it is impossible to say how large is large enough, as it depends on the nature of the particular non-Gaussian distribution. Unless the population distribution is really weird, you are probably safe choosing a parametric test when there are at least two dozen data points in each group.
2. Large sample: What happens when you use a nonparametric test with data from a Gaussian population? Nonparametric tests work well with large samples from Gaussian populations. The P-values tend to be a bit too large, but the discrepancy is small. In other words, nonparametric tests are only slightly less powerful than parametric tests with large samples.
3. Small samples: What happens when you use a parametric test with data from non-Gaussian populations? You cannot rely on the central limit theorem, so the P-value may be inaccurate.
4. Small samples: When you use a nonparametric test with data from a Gaussian population, the P-values tend to be too high. The nonparametric tests lack statistical power with small samples.

Thus, large data sets present no problems. It is usually easy to tell if the data come from a Gaussian population, but it does not really matter because the nonparametric tests are so powerful and the parametric tests are so robust. Small data sets present a dilemma. It is difficult to tell if the data come from a Gaussian population, but it matters a lot. The nonparametric tests are not powerful and the parametric tests are not robust.

EXERCISE

Fill in the blanks:

1. .... tests are used in data which are distributed normally.
2. .... tests are used in the data which are not distributed normally.
3. Nonparametric equivalent of parametric test one way ANOVA is .... test.
4. Parametric equivalent of nonparametric test Mann-Whitney test is .... test.
5. Nominal data follows the .... distribution.
6. There is no need to check the distribution in .... and .... type of data.
7. Measurement of skewness and kurtosis and plotting the histogram are helpful in ....
8. Lateral shifting of normal distribution curve is called ....
9. The value of skewness at both the extreme conditions like extremely right sided skewness and extremely left sided skewness is .... and .... respectively.
10. The value of skewness between .... to .... shows data following the normal distribution.
11. Degree of peakedness relative to the length and size of tails is ....
12. The value of kurtosis between .... to .... show the data are following the normal distribution.
13. Statistical tests to know the distribution of data are .... and ....
14. "Off the scale" values should be analyzed by .... tests.

Answers

1. Parametric
2. Nonparametric
3. Kruskal-Wallis test
4. Unpaired *t* test
5. Chi-square
6. Nominal and ordinal
7. Knowing the distribution of data
8. Skewness
9. +3, –3
10. +1, –1
11. Kurtosis
12. +1, –1
13. Kolmogorov-Smirnov, Shapiro-Wilk
14. Nonparametric tests

Match the following:

1. Parametric test	(a) Test to check the distribution of data
2. Nonparametric test	(b) Data dealing with rank or score
3. Nominal data	(c) Parametric equivalent of Spearman correlation
4. Pearson correlation	(d) Follows Chi-square distribution
5. Wilcoxon test	(e) Distribution should be checked.
6. Skewness	(f) Test for analyzing the data following normal distribution.
7. Kurtosis	(g) Test for analyzing the data which does not follows the normal distribution.
8. Shapiro Wilk test	(h) Nonparametric equivalent of paired *t* test
9. Ordinal data	(i) Amplitude of normal distribution curve
10. Ratio data	(j) Lateral shift of normal distribution curve.

Answers

1. (f)	2. (g)	3. (d)	4. (c)	5. (h)	6. (j)
7. (i)	8. (a)	9. (b)	10. (e)		

True/False exercise (tick the correct):

1. Lateral shift of normal distribution curve is called kurtosis. *True/False*
2. Data of the study having the small sample size (< 30) always follows the normal distribution. *True/False*
3. Komolgorov Smirnov test used to check the distribution of data. *True/False*
4. Ordinal data follows Chi-square distribution. *True/False*
5. Histogram is useful in checking the homogeneity of data. *True/False*
6. Friedman test is nonparametric equivalent of parametric test repeat measure ANOVA. *True/False*
7. Nonparametric tests are used in data which follows the Gaussian distribution. *True/False*
8. Study having the ratio or interval data and sample size is more than 100 usually follows the normal distribution. *True/False*
9. Shapiro-Wilk test is nonparametric equivalent of Kolmogorov-Smirnov test. *True/False*
10. Degree of peakedness relative to the length and size of tails is skewness. *True/False*

Answers

1. False	2. False	3. True	4. False
5. False	6. True	7. False	8. True
9. False	10. False		

Some statistical examples are given below. Read the examples and tick the correct answer from the exercise given with the same.

1. Twenty individuals are chosen from at random from a normal population and there systolic blood pressure in mm Hg are found to be— 110, 112, 140, 120, 124, 122, 142, 110, 126, 132, 134, 114, 144, 160, 140, 124, 122, 146, 152 and 126. Does this sample adequately represent a population in which the mean systolic blood pressure was found to be—140 mm Hg?

Q. For analyzing this data by appropriate statistical test whether the distribution of data should be checked or not? (Tick the correct one).

YES ☐

NO ☐

2. From the data given in table, test whether the prevalence of hypertension, in two different sexes is significantly different.

Sex	*No. with high BP*	*No. without high BP*	*Total*
Male	1168	10200	11368
Female	600	7900	8500
Total	1768	18100	19868

Q. For analyzing this data by appropriate statistical test whether the distribution of data should be checked or not? (Tick the correct one).

YES ☐

NO ☐

3. In a clinical trial to assess the efficacy of new antianxiety drugs on patients of anxiety disorders with each patient

being given a week's treatment with drug. The drug was considered effective if it lowered anxiety score after treatment. Test the efficacy of drug on the following results.

Before treatment—22, 18, 17, 19, 22, 12, 10, 11, 19, 8

After treatment—19, 20, 11, 9, 22, 15, 20, 20, 6, 7

Q. For analyzing this data by appropriate statistical test whether the distribution of data should be checked or not? (Tick the correct one).

YES ☐

NO ☐

Answers

1. YES. Blood pressure is the typical example of the ratio data. Distribution should always be checked in ratio and interval data. As sample size in this example is small (20) so, there are more chances of having non-normal distribution.
2. NO. The data in the question is nominal data. There is no need to check data for distribution in the case of nominal data. These data follow the Chi-square distribution.
3. NO. Here the effect of a new antianxiety drug on anxiety score is evaluated. As we had already discussed that score and ranks are examples of ordinal data (see first Chapter) and there is no need to check distribution in ordinal data as they does not follow the normal distribution. So, straightway nonparametric test should be used in these conditions.

Chapter 4

How to Choose Statistical Test?

Now, we will learn the selection of appropriate statistical test. As we know that two prerequisites of selection of appropriate statistical tests are sound understanding of type of data and ability to check the data for distribution. These prerequisites are already learned by you. Selection of appropriate tests are easy, just you need to understand the following table.

As it can be seen in table, first column deals with the "goal". The goal is the aim of the study. What we want to compare? Whether we want to compare the drug with placebo? Or we want to compare effect of intervention by comparing preintervention endpoints with post-intervention endpoints. Other columns are related to the type of data and distribution of data. Second column is about the ratio and interval data following the normal distribution. So, parametric tests will be used in this type of data. Third column is about the ratio and interval data not following the normal distribution and ordinal data. As we know nonparametric tests will be used during the analysis of these data. Fourth column is about the nominal data. So, if we know the aim of the study, type of data we are dealing with and distribution of data than selection of appropriate statistical test is very easy. Once the appropriate test is selected, we can use any biostatistics software to analyze the data or tests can be performed manually.

	Type of data		
Goal	Ratio and interval data which follows normal distribution	Ratio and interval data which does not follow normal distribution and ordinal data (rank and scores)	Nominal data
Describe one group	Mean, SD	Median, interquartile range	Proportion
Compare one group to a hypothetical value	One-sample *t* test	Wilcoxon test	Chi-square or binomial test
Compare two unpaired groups	Unpaired *t* test	Mann-Whitney test	Fisher's test (Chi-square for large samples)
Compare two paired groups	Paired *t* test	Wilcoxon test	McNemar's test
Compare three or more unmatched groups	One-way ANOVA	Kruskal-Wallis test	Chi-square test
Compare three or more matched groups	Repeated measures ANOVA	Friedman test	Cochrane Q
Quantify association between two variables	Pearson correlation	Spearman correlation	Contingency coefficients
Predict value from another measured variable	Simple linear regression or nonlinear regression	Nonparametric regression	Simple logistic regression
Predict value from several measured or binomial variables	Multiple linear regression or multiple nonlinear regression		Multiple logistic regression

DESCRIBE ONE GROUP

These are the simple parameters to describe a single group. Different groups can be compared on the basis of change in these parameters. Ratio and interval data following the normal distribution are compared on the basis of mean and standard deviation. Usually, these kinds of data are expressed as mean ± standard deviation. The reason why these data are expressed by mean is parametric test compares mean values of variables. In the same way ratio and interval data not following the normal distribution and ordinal data (rank and score) are described by median and range. I suggest that median is better method as range is sensitive to outliers. For analyzing of these data nonparametric tests are used which compares medians of groups. Nominal data are expressed in proportions. It indicates the relationship between the individual events and events in totality. Test for analyzing of nominal data compares the proportions of events between groups.

Example 1: Investigators want to see the effect of a new lipid lowering drug on serum cholesterol. They recruited 100 patients of atherosclerosis. Drug was given for six months. Blood sample for serum cholesterol was taken on day first and after sixth months. Values of serum cholesterol are as follows:

First day—340, 300, 280, 290, 300....................(n-100)
Last day—240, 260, 245, 220..............................(n-100)

Assuming the data follows the normal distribution which is the better method for the description of this group?

Answer

For any exercise related to selection of appropriate statistical test we will ask three basic questions and on the basis of answers of these questions it will be easy to find the appropriate test.

First question: What is the aim?

Here, the aim is to "describe one group".

Second question: What type of data it is?

This is the ratio data as it has meaningful order, absolute zero and equal interval between the measurements.

Third question: Whether the data follow the normal distribution?

In this case data do follow the normal distribution (see question).

In actual analysis of data we are supposed to check the distribution of data by methods explained in previous chapter.

With this much of information see the table for appropriate statistical test. We can see that answer is mean and standard deviation. So "mean" and "standard deviation" are better method for description of this group.

	Type of data		
Goal	Ratio and interval data which follows normal distribution	Ratio and interval data which does not follow normal distribution and ordinal data (rank and scores)	Nominal data
Describe one group	Mean, standard deviation	Median, interquartile range	Proportion
Compare one group to a hypothetical value	One-sample *t* test	Wilcoxon test	Chi-square or binomial test
Compare two unpaired groups	Unpaired *t* test	Mann-Whitney test	Fisher's test (Chi-square for large samples)
Compare two paired groups	Paired *t* test	Wilcoxon test	McNemar's test
Compare three or more unmatched groups	One-way ANOVA	Kruskal-Wallis test	Chi-square test
Compare three or more matched groups	Repeated measures ANOVA	Friedman test	Cochrane Q
Quantify association between two variables	Pearson correlation	Spearman correlation	Contingency coefficients
Predict value from another measured variable	Simple linear regression or nonlinear regression	Nonparametric regression	Simple logistic regression
Predict value from several measured or binomial variables	Multiple linear regression or multiple nonlinear regression		Multiple logistic regression

Example 2: A researcher wants to confirm his hypothesis that medical students are more anxious as compared to engineering students. He selected 50 medical students randomly from medical college and measure there anxiety score. He also selected 50 engineering students from the engineering college and measured the anxiety score. Anxiety scores of both groups are as follows:

Medical students—22, 18, 17, 19......................22 (n-50)

Engineering students—20, 15, 13....................21 (n-50)

Which is the better method for description of this group?

Answer

First question: What is the aim?

Here, the aim is to "describe one group".

Second question: What type of data it is?

Here, anxiety score is measured in both the groups. Whenever the data is related to rank or score then these types of data are ordinal data as they have meaningful order but there is no equal interval between the orders.

Third question: Whether the data follow the normal distribution?

As we know, ordinal data do not follow the normal distribution.

So, after looking at the table we can say that "median" and "range" are better methods.

	Type of data		
Goal	Ratio and interval data which follows normal distribution	Ratio and interval data which does not follow normal distribution and ordinal data (rank and scores)	Nominal data
Describe one group	Mean, standard deviation	Median, interquartile range	Proportion
Compare one group to a hypothetical value	One-sample *t* test	Wilcoxon test	Chi-square or binomial test
Compare two unpaired groups	Unpaired *t* test	Mann-Whitney test	Fisher's test (Chi-square for large samples)
Compare two paired groups	Paired *t* test	Wilcoxon test	McNemar's test
Compare three or more unmatched groups	One-way ANOVA	Kruskal-Wallis test	Chi-square test
Compare three or more matched groups	Repeated measures ANOVA	Friedman test	Cochrane Q
Quantify association between two variables	Pearson correlation	Spearman correlation	Contingency coefficients
Predict value from another measured variable	Simple linear regression or nonlinear regression	Nonparametric regression	Simple logistic regression
Predict value from several measured or binomial variables	Multiple linear regression or multiple nonlinear regression		Multiple logistic regression

Example 3: From a population 50 females using oral contraceptives and 60 females using other contraceptives devices were randomly selected and number of hypertensive cases from both groups was recorded as given below. Test the hypothesis that the proportion of patients with hypertension is the same for two groups.

Type of contraceptive	*Total*	*No. found hypertensive*
Oral	50	8
Other	60	16

Which is the better method for description of this group?

Answer

First question: What is the aim?

Here, the aim is to "describe one group".

Second question: What type of data it is?

Nominal data. Can be counted but cannot be measured.

Third question: Whether the data follow the normal distribution?

Nominal data follow the Chi-square distribution.

So, on the basis of table the "proportion" is better method for description.

	Type of data		
Goal	Ratio and interval data which follows normal distribution	Ratio and interval data which does not follow normal distribution and ordinal data (rank and scores)	Nominal data
Describe one group	Mean, standard deviation	Median, interquartile range	Proportion
Compare one group to a hypothetical value	One-sample *t* test	Wilcoxon test	Chi-square or binomial test
Compare two unpaired groups	Unpaired *t* test	Mann-Whitney test	Fisher's test (Chi-square for large samples)
Compare two paired groups	Paired *t* test	Wilcoxon test	McNemar's test
Compare three or more unmatched groups	One-way ANOVA	Kruskal-Wallis test	Chi-square test
Compare three or more matched groups	Repeated-measures ANOVA	Friedman test	Cochrane Q
Quantify association between two variables	Pearson correlation	Spearman correlation	Contingency coefficients
Predict value from another measured variable	Simple linear regression or nonlinear regression	Nonparametric regression	Simple logistic regression
Predict value from several measured or binomial variables	Multiple linear regression or multiple nonlinear regression		Multiple logistic regression

> Two of the most common descriptive statistics for continuous data are the mean and standard deviation. However, these statistics correctly describe only a "normal" or "Gaussian" distribution of values. By definition, about 68% of the values of a normal distribution are within plus or minus 1 standard deviation of the mean, about 95% are within plus or minus 2 standard deviations, and about 99% are within plus or minus 3 standard deviations. In markedly, non-normal distributions, these relationships are no longer true, so the mean and standard deviation do not communicate the shape of the distribution well. Instead, other measures, such as the median (the 50th percentile: the value dividing the data into an upper and a lower half) and range (usually reported by giving the minimum and maximum values) or interquartile range (usually reported by giving the 25th and the 75th percentiles) are recommended. Although, the mean and standard deviation can be calculated from as few as two data points, these statistics may not describe small samples well. In addition, most biological data are not normally distributed. For these reasons, the median and range or interquartile range should probably be far more common in the medical literature than the mean and standard deviation.

COMPARE ONE GROUP TO A HYPOTHETICAL VALUE

Here, the study population is compared with the hypothetical value. Researcher is interested in knowing the difference of variable in study population and a hypothetical value (from previous studies).

Example 1: The average weight of population of a country X is 72 kg. 100 subjects were randomly selected from country Y and there weight measured. The weights of those 100 subjects are as follows:

56, 73, 60, 89...49 (n-100)

Is there any significant difference between the weights of two populations?

Assume data follow the normal distribution.

Answer

So, which test we should select to analyze this data? We will use the same three questions.

First question: What is the aim?

Here, the aim is to "compare one group to a hypothetical value".

Second question: What type of data it is?

Weight is the ratio data. It has meaningful order, equal interval and absolute zero.

Third question: Whether the data follow the normal distribution?

In the question it is mentioned that data follow the normal distribution.

So, on the basis of table the most appropriate test in this condition will be "one-sample *t* test".

	Type of data		
Goal	Ratio and interval data which follows normal distribution	Ratio and interval data which does not follow normal distribution and ordinal data (rank and scores)	Nominal data
Describe one group	Mean, standard deviation	Median, interquartile range	Proportion
Compare one group to a hypothetical value	One-sample *t* test	Wilcoxon test	Chi-square or binomial test
Compare two unpaired groups	Unpaired *t* test	Mann-Whitney test	Fisher's test (Chi-square for large samples)
Compare two paired groups	Paired *t* test	Wilcoxon test	McNemar's test
Compare three or more unmatched groups	One-way ANOVA	Kruskal-Wallis test	Chi-square test
Compare three or more matched groups	Repeated-measures ANOVA	Friedman test	Cochrane Q
Quantify association between two variables	Pearson correlation	Spearman correlation	Contingency coefficients
Predict value from another measured variable	Simple linear regression or nonlinear regression	Nonparametric regression	Simple logistic regression
Predict value from several measured or binomial variables	Multiple linear regression or multiple nonlinear regression		Multiple logistic regression

Example 2: In a city A, the average number of attacks of malaria was 2.3 per person. A sample of 15 persons drawn from the city B showed the number of attacks of malaria as follows:

1, 2, 1, 3, 1, 1, 2, 4, 1, 2, 2, 1, 1, 3, 1

Is there any significant difference of attack rate of malaria between the two cities?

Answer

First question: What is the aim?

Here, the aim is to "compare one group to a hypothetical value".

Second question: What type of data it is?

Number of attacks of malaria is nominal data.

Third question: Whether the data follow the normal distribution?

Nominal data follow the Chi-square distribution. There is no need to check nominal data for normal distribution.

So, on the basis of table the most appropriate test in this condition will be "Chi-square or binomial test".

	Type of data		
Goal	Ratio and interval data which follows normal distribution	Ratio and interval data which does not follow normal distribution and ordinal data (rank and scores)	Nominal data
Describe one group	Mean, standard deviation	Median, interquartile range	Proportion
Compare one group to a hypothetical value	One-sample *t* test	Wilcoxon test	Chi-square or binomial test
Compare two unpaired groups	Unpaired *t* test	Mann-Whitney test	Fisher's test (Chi-square for large samples)
Compare two paired groups	Paired *t* test	Wilcoxon test	McNemar's test
Compare three or more unmatched groups	One-way ANOVA	Kruskal-Wallis test	Chi-square test
Compare three or more matched groups	Repeated-measures ANOVA	Friedman test	Cochrane Q
Quantify association between two variables	Pearson correlation	Spearman correlation	Contingency coefficients
Predict value from another measured variable	Simple linear regression or nonlinear regression	Nonparametric regression	Simple logistic regression
Predict value from several measured or binomial variables	Multiple linear regression or multiple nonlinear regression		Multiple logistic regression

Example 3: Average IQ level of males of country A is 110. 15 males of country B are selected and IQ level measured. These are:

90. 100. 110, 50, 70, 50, 100, 100, 80, 80, 90, 94, 60, 100, 100, 70, 110

Is there any significant difference in IQ of males of two countries?

Assume that data do not follow the normal distribution.

Answer

First question: What is the aim?

Here, the aim is to "compare one group to a hypothetical value".

Second question: What type of data it is?

As we had discussed, IQ is interval data. It has magnitude, meaningful order, equal difference but no natural zero.

Third question: Whether the data follow the normal distribution?

As it is given in the exercise that data do not follow the normal distribution.

So, on the basis of table the most appropriate test in this condition will be "Wilcoxon test".

	Type of data		
Goal	Ratio and interval data which follows normal distribution	Ratio and interval data which does not follow normal distribution and ordinal data (rank and scores)	Nominal data
Describe one group	Mean, standard deviation	Median, interquartile range	Proportion
Compare one group to a hypothetical value	One-sample *t* test	Wilcoxon test	Chi-square or Binomial test
Compare two unpaired groups	Unpaired *t* test	Mann-Whitney test	Fisher's test (Chi-square for large samples)
Compare two paired groups	Paired *t* test	Wilcoxon test	McNemar's test
Compare three or more unmatched groups	One-way ANOVA	Kruskal-Wallis test	Chi-square test
Compare three or more matched groups	Repeated-measures ANOVA	Friedman test	Cochrane Q
Quantify association between two variables	Pearson correlation	Spearman correlation	Contingency coefficients
Predict value from another measured variable	Simple linear regression or nonlinear regression	Nonparametric regression	Simple logistic regression
Predict value from several measured or binomial variables	Multiple linear regression or multiple nonlinear regression		Multiple logistic regression

COMPARE TWO UNPAIRED GROUPS

Unpaired test are use to compare groups when the individual values are not paired or matched with one another. Like one intervention is done on one group and another done on another group, then both the groups are compared for the study endpoints. For example, one new drug is tested for its antihypertensive activities. One group given the drug and another given placebo and both the groups compared on the basis of there mean blood pressures.

Example 1: Two groups of diabetic people were selected randomly for the study. For one group metformin was given and for other group a new drug was given for 2 months. Their blood sugar levels at the end of two months are as follows:

Blood sugar level in metformin group	*Blood sugar level in new drug group*
200	200
180	200
260	160
320	180
280	170
200	180
180	260
190	160
220	200
180	190

Which drug is better? (Assume that data follow normal distribution).

Answer

First question: What is the aim?

Here, the aim is to "compare two unpaired groups".

Second question: What type of data it is?

Blood sugar is the ratio data.

Third question: Whether the data follow the normal distribution?

As it is given in the exercise that data follow the normal distribution.

So, on the basis of table the most appropriate test in this condition will be "unpaired *t* test".

Unpaired *t* Test Vs Z Test

There are some prerequisites before using unpaired *t* test. These sample should be drawn randomly from the population, data should be either ratio or interval, data should be distributed normally and sample size should be less than 30. In the case of Z test all criteria are similar except sample size, here sample size should be more than 30.

Question: What do you call a tea (t) party with more than 30 people?

Answer: Z party!!!

	Type of data		
Goal	Ratio and interval data which follows normal distribution	Ratio and interval data which does not follow normal distribution and ordinal data (rank and scores)	Nominal data
Describe one group	Mean, standard deviation	Median, interquartile range	Proportion
Compare one group to a hypothetical value	One-sample *t* test	Wilcoxon test	Chi-square or binomial test
Compare two unpaired groups	Unpaired *t* test	Mann-Whitney test	Fisher's test (Chi-square for large samples)
Compare two paired groups	Paired *t* test	Wilcoxon test	McNemar's test
Compare three or more unmatched groups	One-way ANOVA	Kruskal-Wallis test	Chi-square test
Compare three or more matched groups	Repeated-measures ANOVA	Friedman test	Cochrane Q
Quantify association between two variables	Pearson correlation	Spearman correlation	Contingency coefficients
Predict value from another measured variable	Simple linear regression or nonlinear regression	Nonparametric regression	Simple logistic regression
Predict value from several measured or binomial variables	Multiple linear regression or multiple nonlinear regression		Multiple logistic regression

Example 2: The erythrocyte sedimentation rate (mm/hr) of 15 males and 11 females before start of tuberculosis treatment is given below. Is the difference significant? (Assume that data do not follow the normal distribution).

Males	*Females*
65	63
60	84
110	90
84	100
75	90
103	105
125	98
118	93
83	100
75	111
90	125
95	
128	
65	
84	

Answer

First question: What is the aim?

Here, the aim is to "compare two unpaired groups".

Second question: What type of data it is?

ESR is the ratio data.

Third question: Whether the data follow the normal distribution?

As it is given in the exercise that data do not follow the normal distribution.

So, on the basis of table the most appropriate test in this condition will be "Mann-Whitney test".

	Type of data		
Goal	Ratio and interval data which follows normal distribution	Ratio and interval data which does not follow normal distribution and ordinal data (rank and scores)	Nominal data
Describe one group	Mean, standard deviation	Median, interquartile range	Proportion
Compare one group to a hypothetical value	One-sample *t* test	Wilcoxon test	Chi-square or binomial test
Compare two unpaired groups	Unpaired *t* test	Mann-Whitney test	Fisher's test (Chi-square for large samples)
Compare two paired groups	Paired *t* test	Wilcoxon test	McNemar's test
Compare three or more unmatched groups	One-way ANOVA	Kruskal-Wallis test	Chi-square test
Compare three or more matched groups	Repeated-measures ANOVA	Friedman test	Cochrane Q
Quantify association between two variables	Pearson correlation	Spearman correlation	Contingency coefficients
Predict value from another measured variable	Simple linear regression or nonlinear regression	Nonparametric regression	Simple logistic regression
Predict value from several measured or binomial variables	Multiple linear regression or multiple nonlinear regression		Multiple logistic regression

Example 3: In a clinical trial to assess the efficacy of new antianxiety drugs on patients of anxiety disorders, two groups having the patients of anxiety disorder were formed. One group was given new drug and another group was given placebo. Drug was considered effective if it lowered anxiety score after treatment. After two weeks anxiety scores of subjects of both groups were as follows:

New drug group—22, 18, 17, 19, 22, 12, 10, 11, 19, 8

Placebo group—19, 20, 11, 9, 22, 15, 20, 20, 6, 7

Is the new drug better than the placebo?

Answer

First question: What is the aim?

Here, the aim is to "compare two unpaired groups".

Second question: What type of data it is?

Anxiety score is an ordinal data. Ranks and scores are ordinal data.

Third question: Whether the data follow the normal distribution?

As we know ordinal data do not follow the normal distribution.

So, on the basis of table the most appropriate test in this condition will be "Mann-Whitney test".

	Type of data		
Goal	Ratio and interval data which follows normal distribution	Ratio and interval data which does not follow normal distribution and ordinal data (rank and scores)	Nominal data
Describe one group	Mean, standard deviation	Median, interquartile range	Proportion
Compare one group to a hypothetical value	One-sample *t* test	Wilcoxon test	Chi-square or binomial test
Compare two unpaired groups	Unpaired *t* test	Mann-Whitney test	Fisher's test (Chi-square for large samples)
Compare two paired groups	Paired *t* test	Wilcoxon test	McNemar's test
Compare three or more unmatched groups	One-way ANOVA	Kruskal-Wallis test	Chi-square test
Compare three or more matched groups	Repeated-measures ANOVA	Friedman test	Cochrane Q
Quantify association between two variables	Pearson correlation	Spearman correlation	Contingency coefficients
Predict value from another measured variable	Simple linear regression or nonlinear regression	Nonparametric regression	Simple logistic regression
Predict value from several measured or binomial variables	Multiple linear regression or multiple nonlinear regression		Multiple logistic regression

Example 4: Attack rates among the vaccinated and unvaccinated against measles are given below. Prove the protective value of vaccination by analyzing data with the help of suitable statistical test.

Group ↓	*Attacked*	*Not-attacked*	*Total*
Vaccinated	15	85	100
Unvaccinated	25	75	100
Total	40	160	200

Answer

First question: What is the aim?

Here, the aim is to "compare two unpaired groups".

Second question: What type of data it is?

Attacked, not-attacked is a typical nominal data.

Third question: Whether the data follow the normal distribution?

As we know nominal do not follow the normal distribution but Chi-square distribution. There is no need to check distribution in nominal data.

So, on the basis of table the most appropriate test in this condition will be "Fisher's test". (Chi-square test can be used if sample size is large).

	Type of data		
Goal	Ratio and interval data which follows normal distribution	Ratio and interval data which does not follow normal distribution and ordinal data (rank and scores)	Nominal data
Describe one group	Mean, standard deviation	Median, interquartile range	Proportion
Compare one group to a hypothetical value	One-sample *t* test	Wilcoxon test	Chi-square or binomial test
Compare two unpaired groups	Unpaired *t* test	Mann-Whitney test	Fisher's test (Chi-square for large samples)
Compare two paired groups	Paired *t* test	Wilcoxon test	McNemar's test
Compare three or more unmatched groups	One-way ANOVA	Kruskal-Wallis test	Chi-square test
Compare three or more matched groups	Repeated-measures ANOVA	Friedman test	Cochrane Q
Quantify association between two variables	Pearson correlation	Spearman correlation	Contingency coefficients
Predict value from another measured variable	Simple linear regression or nonlinear regression	Nonparametric regression	Simple logistic regression
Predict value from several measured or binomial variables	Multiple linear regression or multiple nonlinear regression		Multiple logistic regression

Fisher's test Vs Chi-square Test

When analyzing contingency tables with two rows and two columns, we can use either Fisher's exact test or the Chi-square test. The Fisher's test is the best choice as it always gives the exact P-value. The Chi-square test is simpler to calculate but yields only an approximate P-value. If we are using the biostatistics software, we should choose Fisher's test unless we prefer the familiarity of the Chi-square test. We should definitely avoid the Chi-square test when the numbers in the contingency table are very small (any number less than about six). When the numbers are larger, the P-values reported by the Chi-square and Fisher's test will be very similar. The Chi-square test calculates approximate P-values, and the Yate's continuity correction is designed to make the approximation better. Without the Yate's correction, the P values are too low. However, the correction goes too far, and the resulting P-value is too high. Statisticians give different recommendations regarding Yate's correction. With large sample sizes, the Yate's correction makes little difference. If we select Fisher's test, the P-value is exact and Yate's correction is not needed.

COMPARE TWO PAIRED GROUPS

Paired tests are use to compare groups when the individual values are paired or matched with one another. This test is applied to paired data of independent observations from one sample only when each individual gives a pair of observations. Select a paired or repeated-measures test when values represent repeated measurements on one subject (before and after an intervention) or measurements on matched subjects. The paired or repeated-measures tests are also appropriate for repeated laboratory experiments run at different times, each with its own control. Paired test should be selected when values in one group are more closely correlated with a specific value in the other group than with random values in the other group. It is only appropriate to select a paired test when the subjects were matched or paired before the data were collected. Paired test should be used in following conditions:

1. To study the contribution of a factor when the observations are made before and after its play, e.g. effect of drug on serum cholesterol, effect of antidepressants on memory and cognition.
2. To compare the effect of two drugs on same sample population by giving the drugs at different time, e.g. to see the effect of two antidepressants on depression. Baseline depression scale is measured than first antidepressants is given for one month, again depression scale measured and after a washout period second antidepressant is given for one month to same sample.
3. To see comparative accuracy of two instruments, e.g. two types of glucometer.
4. To compare the result of two laboratory techniques, e.g. estimation of hemoglobin by two different methods.
5. To compare the observation made at different part of same body. Temperature measurement at axilla and mouth.

Example 1: Systolic blood pressure of 10 hypertensive individuals who had been recumbent for 5 minutes was taken. Then 2 ml of new antihypertensive drug was given through parentral route and blood pressure is recorded again. Did the injection of drug lower the blood pressure? (Assume the data follow the normal distribution).

Blood pressure before injection—146, 150, 160, 166, 180, 150, 170, 184, 152

Blood pressure after injection—120, 132, 140, 164, 170, 160, 134, 142, 150

Answer

First question: What is the aim?

Here, the aim is to "compare two paired groups"

Second question: What type of data it is?

Blood pressure is a ratio data.

Third question: Whether the data follow the normal distribution?

As it is given in the exercise data follow the normal distribution.

So, on the basis of table the most appropriate test in this condition will be "Paired t test".

	Type of data		
Goal	Ratio and interval data which follows normal distribution	Ratio and interval data which does not follow normal distribution and ordinal data (rank and scores)	Nominal data
Describe one group	Mean, standard deviation	Median, interquartile range	Proportion
Compare one group to a hypothetical value	One-sample *t* test	Wilcoxon test	Chi-square or binomial test
Compare two unpaired groups	Unpaired *t* test	Mann-Whitney test	Fisher's test (Chi-square for large samples)
Compare two paired groups	Paired *t* test	Wilcoxon test	McNemar's test
Compare three or more unmatched groups	One-way ANOVA	Kruskal-Wallis test	Chi-square test
Compare three or more matched groups	Repeated-measures ANOVA	Friedman test	Cochrane Q
Quantify association between two variables	Pearson correlation	Spearman correlation	Contingency coefficients
Predict value from another measured variable	Simple linear regression or nonlinear regression	Nonparametric regression	Simple logistic regression Multiple logistic regression
Predict value from several measured or binomial variables	Multiple linear regression or multiple nonlinear regression		

Example 2: In a clinical trial to assess the efficacy of new antianxiety drugs on patients of anxiety disorders with each patient being given a week's treatment with drug. The drug was considered effective if it lowered anxiety score after treatment. Test the efficacy of drug on the following results:

Before treatment—22, 18, 17, 19, 22, 12, 10, 11, 19, 8

After treatment—19, 20, 11, 9, 22, 15, 20, 20, 6, 7

Answer

First question: What is the aim?

Here, the aim is to "compare two paired groups".

Second question: What type of data it is?

Anxiety score is an ordinal data.

Third question: Whether the data follow the normal distribution?

Ordinal data do not follow the normal distribution.

So, on the basis of table the most appropriate test in this condition will be "Wilcoxon test".

	Type of data		
Goal	Ratio and interval data which follows normal distribution	Ratio and interval data which does not follow normal distribution and ordinal data (rank and scores)	Nominal data
Describe one group	Mean, standard deviation	Median, interquartile range	Proportion
Compare one group to a hypothetical value	One-sample *t* test	Wilcoxon test	Chi-square or binomial test
Compare two unpaired groups	Unpaired *t* test	Mann-Whitney test	Fisher's test (Chi-square for large samples)
Compare two paired groups	Paired *t* test	Wilcoxon test	McNemar's test
Compare three or more unmatched groups	One-way ANOVA	Kruskal-Wallis test	Chi-square test
Compare three or more matched groups	Repeated-measures ANOVA	Friedman test	Cochrane Q
Quantify association between two variables	Pearson correlation	Spearman correlation	Contingency coefficients
Predict value from another measured variable	Simple linear regression or nonlinear regression	Nonparametric regression	Simple logistic regression
Predict value from several measured or binomial variables	Multiple linear regression or multiple nonlinear regression		Multiple logistic regression

Example 3: The weight of 9 tuberculosis patients on admission and at the end of 12 months of treatment with pyrazinamide plus isoniazid daily, are given below. Examine whether the gain in weight is statistically significant.

Weight on admission (kg)	*Weight after 12 months (kg)*
49	52
41	50
37	42
42	40
41	51
36	43
35	44
38	39
43	53

Assume that data does not distributed normally.

Answer

First question: What is the aim?

Here, the aim is to "compare two paired groups".

Second question: What type of data it is?

Weight is a ratio data.

Third question: Whether the data follow the normal distribution?

It is given in the exercise that they are not distributed normally.

So, on the basis of table the most appropriate test in this condition will be "Wilcoxon test".

	Type of data		
Goal	Ratio and interval data which follows normal distribution	Ratio and interval data which does not follow normal distribution and ordinal data (rank and scores)	Nominal data
Describe one group	Mean, standard deviation	Median, interquartile range	Proportion
Compare one group to a hypothetical value	One-sample *t* test	Wilcoxon test	Chi-square or binomial test
Compare two unpaired groups	Unpaired *t* test	Mann-Whitney test	Fisher's test (Chi-square for large samples)
Compare two paired groups	Paired *t* test	Wilcoxon test	McNemar's test
Compare three or more unmatched groups	One-way ANOVA	Kruskal-Wallis test	Chi-square test
Compare three or more matched groups	Repeated-measures ANOVA	Friedman test	Cochrane Q
Quantify association between two variables	Pearson correlation	Spearman correlation	Contingency coefficients
Predict value from another measured variable	Simple linear regression or nonlinear regression	Nonparametric regression	Simple logistic regression
Predict value from several measured or binomial variables	Multiple linear regression or multiple nonlinear regression		Multiple logistic regression

Example 4: To see the allergic potential of a new drug A, a researcher compared it with an established drug for same indication, drug B. She selected 10 subjects and drug A administered and sign and symptoms of allergy is observed. After a week she administered drug B to same 10 subjects and observed the sign and symptom of allergy. Data of the study are given below. Which drug is having less allergy potential?

Serial No. of subjects	*Allergy observed in drug A*	*Allergy observed in drug B*
1	Yes	No
2	No	No
3	No	No
4	Yes	No
5	Yes	Yes
6	No	No
7	No	No
8	No	No
9	No	No
10	Yes	No

Answer

First question: What is the aim?

Here, the aim is to "compare two paired groups".

Second question: What type of data it is?

This is a nominal data.

Third question: Whether the data follow the normal distribution?

Nominal data do not follow the normal distribution.

So, on the basis of table the most appropriate test in this condition will be "McNemar's test".

	Type of data		
Goal	Ratio and interval data which follows normal distribution	Ratio and interval data which does not follow normal distribution and ordinal data (rank and scores)	Nominal data
Describe one group	Mean, standard deviation	Median, interquartile range	Proportion
Compare one group to a hypothetical value	One-sample *t* test	Wilcoxon test	Chi-square or binomial test
Compare two unpaired groups	Unpaired *t* test	Mann-Whitney test	Fisher's test (Chi-square for large samples)
Compare two paired groups	Paired *t* test	Wilcoxon test	McNemar's test
Compare three or more unmatched groups	One-way ANOVA	Kruskal-Wallis test	Chi-square test
Compare three or more matched groups	Repeated-measures ANOVA	Friedman test	Cochrane Q
Quantify association between two variables	Pearson correlation	Spearman correlation	Contingency coefficients
Predict value from another measured variable	Simple linear regression or nonlinear regression	Nonparametric regression	Simple logistic regression
Predict value from several measured or binomial variables	Multiple linear regression or multiple nonlinear regression		Multiple logistic regression

COMPARE THREE OR MORE UNMATCHED GROUPS

When groups are three or more than three then inspite of using "unpaired" or "paired" terminology, "unmatched" and "matched" is used.

Example 1: A researcher wants to see the effect of four new herbs on hemoglobin level. She selected 7 subjects in each group. A fixed dose of four herbs is given to there respective group for one month. Is there any significant difference in the hemoglobin level between the groups? (Assume the data follow normal distribution).

Subjects	*Hb (gm %) Herb A*	*Hb (gm %) Herb B*	*Hb (gm %) Herb C*	*Hb (gm %) Herb D*
1	10.2	11.7	10.8	12.1
2	11.0	10.1	11.3	11.8
3	9.8	9.7	12.1	11.2
4	12.4	11.4	11.6	12.7
5	11.6	10.6	12.2	13.2
6	13.1	10.3	10.9	14.1
7	10.5	11.9	12.5	13.4

Answer

First question: What is the aim?

Here, the aim is to "compare three or more unmatched groups".

Second question: What type of data it is?

Hemoglobin is a ratio data.

Third question: Whether the data follow the normal distribution?

As it is given in the question, data follow the normal distribution.

So, on the basis of table the most appropriate test in this condition will be "One-way ANOVA".

	Type of data		
Goal	Ratio and interval data which follow normal distribution	Ratio and interval data which does not follow normal distribution and ordinal data (rank and scores)	Nominal data
Describe one group	Mean, standard deviation	Median, interquartile range	Proportion
Compare one group to a hypothetical value	One-sample *t* test	Wilcoxon test	Chi-square or binomial test
Compare two unpaired groups	Unpaired *t* test	Mann-Whitney test	Fisher's test (Chi-square for large samples)
Compare two paired groups	Paired *t* test	Wilcoxon test	McNemar's test
Compare three or more unmatched groups	One-way ANOVA	Kruskal-Wallis test	Chi-square test
Compare three or more matched groups	Repeated-measures ANOVA	Friedman test	Cochrane Q
Quantify association between two variables	Pearson correlation	Spearman correlation	Contingency coefficients
Predict value from another measured variable	Simple linear regression or nonlinear regression	Nonparametric regression	Simple logistic regression
Predict value from several measured or binomial variables	Multiple linear regression or multiple nonlinear regression		Multiple logistic regression

Analysis of Covariance (ANCOVA)

Analysis of covariance is a more sophisticated method of analysis of variance. It is based on inclusion of supplementary variables (covariates) into the model. This lets you account for inter-group variation associated not with the "treatment" itself, but with covariate(s). Suppose you analyze the results of a clinical trial of three types of treatment of a disease—"Placebo", "Drug 1", and "Drug 2". The results are three sets of survival times, corresponding to patients from the three treatment groups. The question of interest is whether there is a difference between the three types of treatment in the average survival time. You might use analysis of variance to answer this question. But, if you have supplementary information, for example, each patient's age, then analysis of covariance allows you to adjust the treatment effect (survival time, in this case) to a particular age, say, the mean age of all patients. Age in this case is a "covariate" — it is not related to treatment, but can affect the survival time. This adjustment allows you to reduce the observed variation between the three groups caused not by the treatment itself but by variation of age. If the covariate(s) are associated with the treatment effect, then analysis of covariance may have more power than analysis of variance.

Example 2: Systolic blood pressure values of three occupations are given. Determine if there is any significant difference in mean systolic blood pressure of three groups. (Assume the data does not follow normal distribution).

SBP (mm Hg) Officers group	*SBP (mm Hg) Clerks group*	*SBP (mm Hg) Peons group*
130	125	156
134	136	123
124	154	180
115	122	142
125	160	120
156	180	162
135	118	166
140	112	170
120	142	123
122	124	134

Answer

First question: What is the aim?

Here, the aim is to "compare three or more unmatched groups".

Second question: What type of data it is?

Blood pressure is a ratio data.

Third question: Whether the data follow the normal distribution?

As it is given in the question, data do not follow the normal distribution.

So, on the basis of table the most appropriate test in this condition will be "Kruskal-Wallis test".

	Type of data		
Goal	Ratio and interval data which follows normal distribution	Ratio and interval data which does not follow normal distribution and ordinal data (rank and scores)	Nominal data
Describe one group	Mean, standard deviation	Median, interquartile range	Proportion
Compare one group to a hypothetical value	One-sample *t* test	Wilcoxon test	Chi-square or binomial test
Compare two unpaired groups	Unpaired *t* test	Mann-Whitney test	Fisher's test (Chi-square for large samples)
Compare two paired groups	Paired *t* test	Wilcoxon test	McNemar's test
Compare three or more unmatched groups	One-way ANOVA	Kruskal-Wallis test	Chi-square test
Compare three or more matched groups	Repeated-measures ANOVA	Friedman test	Cochrane Q
Quantify association between two variables	Pearson correlation	Spearman correlation	Contingency coefficients
Predict value from another measured variable	Simple linear regression or nonlinear regression	Nonparametric regression	Simple logistic regression
Predict value from several measured or binomial variables	Multiple linear regression or multiple nonlinear regression		Multiple logistic regression

Example 3: A pharmacologist wants to see the effect of a new antianxiety drug "N". She wants to compare this new drug with an established drug alprazolam and Placebo. She recruited 10 patients of anxiety in each group by simple randomization. Drugs and placebo were given for 2 months. The anxiety score of all the three groups are given below. Is there any difference between the outcomes in three groups?

Anxiety scores "N"	Anxiety score *Alprazolam*	Anxiety score *Placebo*
22	11	20
18	9	15
15	11	14
16	12	17
20	15	20
15	22	16
14	12	15
14	15	14
11	15	12
11	10	10

Answer

First question: What is the aim?

Here, the aim is to "compare three or more unmatched groups".

Second question: What type of data it is?

This data is an ordinal data.

Third question: Whether the data follow the normal distribution?

Ordinal data do not follow the normal distribution.

So, on the basis of table the most appropriate test in this condition will be "Kruskal-Wallis test".

	Type of data		
Goal	Ratio and interval data which follows normal distribution	Ratio and interval data which does not follow normal distribution and ordinal data (rank and scores)	Nominal data
Describe one group	Mean, standard deviation	Median, interquartile range	Proportion
Compare one group to a hypothetical value	One-sample *t* test	Wilcoxon test	Chi-square or binomial test
Compare two unpaired groups	Unpaired *t* test	Mann-Whitney test	Fisher's test (Chi-square for large samples)
Compare two paired groups	Paired *t* test	Wilcoxon test	McNemar's test
Compare three or more unmatched groups	One-way ANOVA	Kruskal-Wallis test	Chi-square test
Compare three or more matched groups	Repeated-measures ANOVA	Friedman test	Cochrane Q
Quantify association between two variables	Pearson correlation	Spearman correlation	Contingency coefficients
Predict value from another measured variable	Simple linear regression or nonlinear regression	Nonparametric regression	Simple logistic regression
Predict value from several measured or binomial variables	Multiple linear regression or multiple nonlinear regression		Multiple logistic regression

Example 4: In order to examine the effect of sedatives and stimulants on driving skills, 150 people selected at random were given either a stimulant, sedative or an identically appearing placebo. After receiving the medication, the participants were administered a battery of coordination and reaction time tests and number of mistakes for each was recorded. Based on this data, can it be concluded that proportion of mistakes is different in three groups?

Medication	*Total number of mistakes*			*Total*
	0-5	*6-10*	*11-15*	
Stimulant	10	20	20	50
Sedative	5	15	30	50
Placebo	25	15	10	50
	40	50	60	150

Answer

First question: What is the aim?

Here, the aim is to "compare three or more unmatched groups".

Second question: What type of data it is?

This data is nominal data (you can count but cannot measure).

Third question: Whether the data follow the normal distribution?

Nominal data do not follow the normal distribution. So, on the basis of table the most appropriate test in this condition will be "Chi-square test".

	Type of data		
Goal	Ratio and interval data which follows normal distribution	Ratio and interval data which does not follow normal distribution and ordinal data (rank and scores)	Nominal data
Describe one group	Mean, standard deviation	Median, interquartile range	Proportion
Compare one group to a hypothetical value	One-sample *t* test	Wilcoxon test	Chi-square or binomial test
Compare two unpaired groups	Unpaired *t* test	Mann-Whitney test	Fisher's test (Chi-square for large samples)
Compare two paired groups	Paired *t* test	Wilcoxon test	McNemar's test
Compare three or more unmatched groups	One-way ANOVA	Kruskal-Wallis test	Chi-square test
Compare three or more matched groups	Repeated-measures ANOVA	Friedman test	Cochrane Q
Quantify association between two variables	Pearson correlation	Spearman correlation	Contingency coefficients
Predict value from another measured variable	Simple linear regression or nonlinear regression	Nonparametric regression	Simple logistic regression
Predict value from several measured or binomial variables	Multiple linear regression or multiple nonlinear regression		Multiple logistic regression

COMPARE THREE OR MORE MATCHED GROUPS

Here, the groups are either three or more than three but they are paired or matched with each other.

Example 1: Following data pertain to the experiment for testing 4 antidiabetic drugs for their action in reducing blood sugar levels. Each drug is given to the each of the 6 patients of diabetes. The order in which a subject was administered a given drug was randomized. A sufficient time was also allowed between the administrations of test of drugs to avoid the effect of one test material upon the subsequent test materials. Is there any significant difference in outcome between all the four groups? Assume data follow the normal distribution.

Patients	*Blood sugar level*			
	Drug A	*Drug B*	*Drug C*	*Drug D*
1	92	109	81	118
2	101	117	94	127
3	88	100	97	106
4	78	99	89	104
5	85	106	79	110
6	98	114	87	126

Answer

First question: What is the aim?

Here, the aim is to "compare three or more matched groups".

Second question: What type of data it is?

Blood sugar is a ratio data.

Third question: Whether the data follow the normal distribution?

Data follow the normal distribution (given in exercise) So, on the basis of table the most appropriate test in this condition will be "repeated-measures ANOVA".

	Type of data		
Goal	Ratio and interval data which follows normal distribution	Ratio and interval data which does not follow normal distribution and ordinal data (rank and scores)	Nominal data
Describe one group	Mean, standard deviation	Median, interquartile range	Proportion
Compare one group to a hypothetical value	One-sample *t* test	Wilcoxon test	Chi-square or binomial test
Compare two unpaired groups	Unpaired *t* test	Mann-Whitney test	Fisher's test (Chi-square for large samples)
Compare two paired groups	Paired *t* test	Wilcoxon test	McNemar's test
Compare three or more unmatched groups	One-way ANOVA	Kruskal-Wallis test	Chi-square test
Compare three or more matched groups	Repeated-measures ANOVA	Friedman test	Cochrane Q
Quantify association between two variables	Pearson correlation	Spearman correlation	Contingency coefficients
Predict value from another measured variable	Simple linear regression or nonlinear regression	Nonparametric regression	Simple logistic regression
Predict value from several measured or binomial variables	Multiple linear regression or multiple nonlinear regression		Multiple logistic regression

Example 2: Details of 20 matched subjects who were on treatment with varieties of multiple vitamins and minerals for improving weight (in kg) are given below. Is there any significant difference in treatment outcome between the groups? (Assume that the data do not follow the normal distribution).

Subjects	*Treatment groups*				
	1	*2*	*3*	*4*	*5*
1	60.1	65.1	63.1	64.0	62.1
2	62.0	65.2	61.2	67.0	65.4
3	61.1	68.0	61.3	63.0	62.2
4	60.2	65.3	60.3	61.4	64.1

Answer

First question: What is the aim?

Here, the aim is to "compare three or more matched groups" (do not confuse the table as unpaired data as all the groups are matched with each other so tests for matched group will be used).

Second question: What type of data it is?

Weight is a ratio data.

Third question: Whether the data follow the normal distribution?

Data do not follow the normal distribution (given in exercise) So, on the basis of table the most appropriate test in this condition will be "Friedman test".

	Type of data		
Goal	Ratio and interval data which follows normal distribution	Ratio and interval data which does not follow normal distribution and ordinal data (rank and scores)	Nominal data
Describe one group	Mean, standard deviation	Median, interquartile range	Proportion
Compare one group to a hypothetical value	One-sample *t* test	Wilcoxon test	Chi-square or binomial test
Compare two unpaired groups	Unpaired *t* test	Mann-Whitney test	Fisher's test (Chi-square for large samples)
Compare two paired groups	Paired *t* test	Wilcoxon test	McNemar's test
Compare three or more unmatched groups	One-way ANOVA	Kruskal-Wallis test	Chi-square test
Compare three or more matched groups	Repeated-measures ANOVA	Friedman test	Cochrane Q
Quantify association between two variables	Pearson correlation	Spearman correlation	Contingency coefficients
Predict value from another measured variable	Simple linear regression or nonlinear regression	Nonparametric regression	Simple logistic regression
Predict value from several measured or binomial variables	Multiple linear regression or multiple nonlinear regression		Multiple logistic regression

Example 3: Pain scores of five patients each receiving four separate treatments. Is there any significant difference between the groups?

Patients	*Treatments*			
	A	*B*	*C*	*D*
1	6	9	10	16
2	9	16	16	32
3	14	14	22	67
4	10	14	40	19
5	11	16	17	60

Answer

First question: What is the aim?

Here, the aim is to "compare three or more matched groups" (in this example four different treatments are given to same set of five patients).

Second question: What type of data it is?

Pain score is an ordinal data.

Third question: Whether the data follow the normal distribution?

Ordinal data do not follow the normal distribution

So, on the basis of table the most appropriate test in this condition will be "Friedman test".

	Type of data		
Goal	Ratio and interval data which follows normal distribution	Ratio and interval data which does not follow normal distribution and ordinal data (rank and scores)	Nominal data
Describe one group	Mean, standard deviation	Median, interquartile range	Proportion
Compare one group to a hypothetical value	One-sample *t* test	Wilcoxon test	Chi-square or binomial test
Compare two unpaired groups	Unpaired *t* test	Mann-Whitney test	Fisher's test (Chi-square for large samples)
Compare two paired groups	Paired *t* test	Wilcoxon test	McNemar's test
Compare three or more unmatched groups	One-way ANOVA	Kruskal-Wallis test	Chi-square test
Compare three or more matched groups	Repeated-measures ANOVA	Friedman test	Cochrane Q
Quantify association between two variables	Pearson correlation	Spearman correlation	Contingency coefficients
Predict value from another measured variable	Simple linear regression or nonlinear regression	Nonparametric regression	Simple logistic regression
Predict value from several measured or binomial variables	Multiple linear regression or multiple nonlinear regression		Multiple logistic regression

Example 4: Four different drugs were given to 20 matched patients (four group containing five patient each) of a particular disease. Those who were cured labeled as 1 and those who were not cured were labeled as 0. Determine by the use of suitable statistical test if there is any significant difference between four groups.

Patients	*Drugs*			
	A	*B*	*C*	*D*
1	1	0	0	1
2	0	1	1	1
3	0	1	0	1
4	0	1	0	1
5	1	0	0	0

Answer

First question: What is the aim?

Here, the aim is to "compare three or more matched groups".

Second question: What type of data it is?

This is a nominal data (cured/not cured).

Third question: Whether the data follow the normal distribution?

Nominal data do not follow the normal distribution

So, on the basis of table the most appropriate test in this condition will be "Cochrane Q".

	Type of data		
Goal	Ratio and interval data which follows normal distribution	Ratio and interval data which does not follow normal distribution and ordinal data (rank and scores)	Nominal data
Describe one group	Mean, standard deviation	Median, interquartile range	Proportion
Compare one group to a hypothetical value	One-sample *t* test	Wilcoxon test	Chi-square or binomial test
Compare two unpaired groups	Unpaired *t* test	Mann-Whitney test	Fisher's test (Chi-square for large samples)
Compare two paired groups	Paired *t* test	Wilcoxon test	McNemar's test
Compare three or more unmatched groups	One-way ANOVA	Kruskal-Wallis test	Chi-square test
Compare three or more matched groups	Repeated-measures ANOVA	Friedman test	Cochrane Q
Quantify association between two variables	Pearson correlation	Spearman correlation	Contingency coefficients
Predict value from another measured variable	Simple linear regression or nonlinear regression	Nonparametric regression	Simple logistic regression
Predict value from several measured or binomial variables	Multiple linear regression or multiple nonlinear regression		Multiple logistic regression

Quantify Association Between Two Variables

We quantify association between two variables by correlation. It determines association between two variables but does not suggest the causality (see tests for causation given below). The extent of correlation ranges between –1 to +1. Aging and blood pressure, intake of calories and proteins, economical status and health status etc. are some example of correlations.

Example 1: During an experiment muscular contraction of guinea pig ileum muscle were measured against different doses of a given drug. The height of curve was considered as the response to the drug. The observations were as below:

Serial No. of experiments	*Dose of drug (µg/ml)*	*Response to drug (mm)*
1	0.3	54.0
2	0.4	59.0
3	0.6	60.0
4	0.8	65.0
5	0.9	70.0

Is there any significant association between two variables? (Assume normal distribution).

Answer

First question: What is the aim?

Here, the aim is to "quantify association between two variables".

Second question: What type of data it is?

Drug dose and response both are ratio data.

Third question: Whether the data follow the normal distribution?

Data follow the normal distribution (given in exercise).

So, on the basis of table the most appropriate test in this condition will be "Pearson correlation".

Assumptions which need to be followed for calculation of Pearson's coefficient (r-value)

1. Data should be normally distributed
2. Two variables should be strictly independent
3. Only single pair of measurement should be made on each subject
4. Every r-value should be accompanied by P-value and confidence interval.

	Type of data		
Goal	Ratio and interval data which follows normal distribution	Ratio and interval data which does not follow normal distribution and ordinal data (rank and scores)	Nominal data
Describe one group	Mean, standard deviation	Median, interquartile range	Proportion
Compare one group to a hypothetical value	One-sample *t* test	Wilcoxon test	Chi-square or binomial test
Compare two unpaired groups	Unpaired *t* test	Mann-Whitney test	Fisher's test (Chi-square for large samples)
Compare two paired groups	Paired *t* test	Wilcoxon test	McNemar's test
Compare three or more unmatched groups	One-way ANOVA	Kruskal-Wallis test	Chi-square test
Compare three or more matched groups	Repeated-measures ANOVA	Friedman test	Cochrane Q
Quantify association between two variables	Pearson correlation	Spearman correlation	Contingency coefficients
Predict value from another measured variable	Simple linear regression or nonlinear regression	Nonparametric regression	Simple logistic regression
Predict value from several measured or binomial variables	Multiple linear regression or multiple nonlinear regression		Multiple logistic regression

Example 2: In the table below gain in weight and gain in height of 8 children in a particular observation period is given. Is there any significant association between two variables? (Data do not follow the normal distribution).

Child number	*Gain in weight (kg)*	*Gain in height (cm)*
1	1	2
2	3	3.5
3	2.5	3
4	4.5	5
5	1.5	2
6	2.0	2.5
7	3.1	3.6
8	4.1	3.8

Answer

First question: What is the aim?

Here, the aim is to "quantify association between two variables".

Second question: What type of data it is?

Weight and height both are the ratio data.

Third question: Whether the data follow the normal distribution?

Data do not follow the normal distribution (given in exercise). So, on the basis of table the most appropriate test in this condition will be "Spearman correlation".

	Type of data		
Goal	Ratio and interval data which follows normal distribution	Ratio and interval data which does not follow normal distribution and ordinal data (rank and scores)	Nominal data
Describe one group	Mean, standard deviation	Median, interquartile range	Proportion
Compare one group to a hypothetical value	One-sample *t* test	Wilcoxon test	Chi-square or binomial test
Compare two unpaired groups	Unpaired *t* test	Mann-Whitney test	Fisher's test (Chi-square for large samples)
Compare two paired groups	Paired *t* test	Wilcoxon test	McNemar's test
Compare three or more unmatched groups	One-way ANOVA	Kruskal-Wallis test	Chi-square test
Compare three or more matched groups	Repeated-measures ANOVA	Friedman test	Cochrane Q
Quantify association between two variables	Pearson correlation	Spearman correlation	Contingency coefficients
Predict value from another measured variable	Simple linear regression or nonlinear regression	Nonparametric regression	Simple logistic regression
Predict value from several measured or binomial variables	Multiple linear regression or multiple nonlinear regression		Multiple logistic regression

Example 3: Calculate the association between grades of smoking and severity of cancer.

Individuals and ranks	*Grades of smoking*	*Severity of cancer*
1	1	2
2	2	1
3	3	4
4	4	3
5	5	6
6	6	7
7	7	5
8	8	9
9	9	8
10	10	10

Answer

First question: What is the aim?

Here, the aim is to "quantify association between two variables".

Second question: What type of data it is?

These data are ordinal data (rank and scores are ordinal data).

Third question: Whether the data follow the normal distribution?

Ordinal data do not follow the normal distribution.So, on the basis of table the most appropriate test in this condition will be "Spearman correlation".

	Type of data		
Goal	Ratio and interval data which follows normal distribution	Ratio and interval data which does not follow normal distribution and ordinal data (rank and scores)	Nominal data
Describe one group	Mean, standard deviation	Median, interquartile range	Proportion
Compare one group to a hypothetical value	One-sample *t* test	Wilcoxon test	Chi-square or binomial test
Compare two unpaired groups	Unpaired *t* test	Mann-Whitney test	Fisher's test (Chi-square for large samples)
Compare two paired groups	Paired *t* test	Wilcoxon test	McNemar's test
Compare three or more unmatched groups	One-way ANOVA	Kruskal-Wallis test	Chi-square test
Compare three or more matched groups	Repeated-measures ANOVA	Friedman test	Cochrane Q
Quantify association between two variables	Pearson correlation	Spearman correlation	Contingency coefficients
Predict value from another measured variable	Simple linear regression or nonlinear regression	Nonparametric regression	Simple logistic regression
Predict value from several measured or binomial variables	Multiple linear regression or multiple nonlinear regression		Multiple logistic regression

Example 4: To see the association of a genetic disease with race, 15 subjects of different race are selected. They are labeled as 1 for American, 2 for oriental and 3 for African. The presence of disease labeled as 1 and absence of disease labeled as 0. Determine whether disease is associated with some race?

Subjects	*Race*	*Disease*
1	1	0
2	3	1
3	1	1
4	2	0
5	3	1
6	1	1
7	3	0
8	2	0
9	2	0
10	3	0
11	1	1
12	2	1
13	2	0
14	1	0
15	3	0

Answer

First question: What is the aim?

Here, the aim is to "quantify association between two variables".

Second question: What type of data it is?

These data are nominal data.

Third question: Whether the data follow the normal distribution?

Nominal data does not follow the normal distribution

So, on the basis of table the most appropriate test in this condition will be "contingency coefficients".

Tests for Causations

To establish the causation these criteria need to be fulfilled:

1. Is there evidence from true experiments in human?
2. Is the association consistent from study to study?
3. Is the temporal relation appropriate?
4. Is there dose response gradient?
5. Does the association make epidemiological sense?
6. Does the association make biological sense?
7. Is the association specific?
8. Is the association analogous to a previously proved causal association?

	Type of data		
Goal	Ratio and interval data which follows normal distribution	Ratio and interval data which does not follow normal distribution and ordinal data (rank and scores)	Nominal data
Describe one group	Mean, standard deviation	Median, interquartile range	Proportion
Compare one group to a hypothetical value	One-sample *t* test	Wilcoxon test	Chi-square or binomial test
Compare two unpaired groups	Unpaired *t* test	Mann-Whitney test	Fisher's test (Chi-square for large samples)
Compare two paired groups	Paired *t* test	Wilcoxon test	McNemar's test
Compare three or more unmatched groups	One-way ANOVA	Kruskal-Wallis test	Chi-square test
Compare three or more matched groups	Repeated-measures ANOVA	Friedman test	Cochrane Q
Quantify association between two variables	Pearson correlation	Spearman correlation	Contingency coefficients
Predict value from another measured variable	Simple linear regression or nonlinear regression	Nonparametric regression	Simple logistic regression
Predict value from several measured or binomial variables	Multiple linear regression or multiple nonlinear regression		Multiple logistic regression

PREDICT VALUE FROM ANOTHER MEASURED VARIABLE

It can be done by regression analysis. Regression analysis is any statistical method where the mean of one or more random variables is predicted based on other measured random variables. There are two types of regression analysis, chosen according to whether the data approximate a straight line, when linear regression is used or not, when non-linear regression is used. A regression line is a line drawn through a scatter plot of two variables. The line is chosen so that, it comes as close to the points as possible. Regression analysis, on the other hand, is more than curve fitting. It involves fitting a model with both deterministic and stochastic components. The deterministic component is called the predictor and the stochastic component is called the error term. The simplest form of a regression model contains a dependent variable, also called the "Y-variable" and a single independent variable, also called the "X-variable". Some examples of the regression of Y on X are the dependence of the blood pressure Y on the age X of a person and the dependence of the weight Y of certain animals on their daily ration of food X.

Example 1: A random group of 10 father-son pair selected and there height measured. We would like to know whether there is any linear or nonlinear relationship between the heights of fathers and sons and we would like to predict height of father on the basis of height of son, i.e. if son's height is 72 inch, what will be the height of the father (Assume normal distribution of data).

Serial No.	*Height (inches)*	
	Adult son (y)	*Father (x)*
1	68	65
2	66	63
3	68	67
4	65	64
5	69	68
6	66	62
7	68	70
8	65	66
9	71	68
10	67	67

Answer

First question: What is the aim?

Here, the aim is to "predict value from another measured variable".

Second question: What type of data it is?

These data are ratio data.

Third question: Whether the data follow the normal distribution?

Data follow the normal distribution (see exercise).

So, on the basis of table the most appropriate test in this condition will be "simple linear regression or nonlinear regression".

> Every scientific article that includes a statistical analysis should contain a sentence confirming that the assumptions on which the analysis is based were met. This confirmation is especially important in linear regression analysis, which assumes that the relationship between a response and an explanatory variable is linear. If this assumption is not met, the results of the analysis may be incorrect. The assumption of linearity may be tested by graphing the "residuals": the difference between each data point and the regression line. If this graph is flat and close to zero, the relationship is linear. If the graph shows any other pattern, the relationship is not linear. Testing the assumption of linearity is important because simply looking at graphed data can be misleading.

	Type of data		
Goal	Ratio and interval data which follows normal distribution	Ratio and interval data which does not follow normal distribution and ordinal data (rank and scores)	Nominal data
Describe one group	Mean, standard deviation	Median, interquartile range	Proportion
Compare one group to a hypothetical value	One-sample *t* test	Wilcoxon test	Chi-square or binomial test
Compare two unpaired groups	Unpaired *t* test	Mann-Whitney test	Fisher's test (Chi-square for large samples)
Compare two paired groups	Paired *t* test	Wilcoxon test	McNemar's test
Compare three or more unmatched groups	One-way ANOVA	Kruskal-Wallis test	Chi-square test
Compare three or more matched groups	Repeated-measures ANOVA	Friedman test	Cochrane Q
Quantify association between two variables	Pearson correlation	Spearman correlation	Contingency coefficients
Predict value from another measured variable	Simple linear regression or nonlinear regression	Nonparametric regression	Simple logistic regression
Predict value from several measured or binomial variables	Multiple linear regression or multiple nonlinear regression		Multiple logistic regression

Example 2: During laboratory experiment muscular contraction of a isolated tissue were measured against different doses of drug. The height of curve considered as response to drug. The observations were as below. What will be the response of tissue at the dose of 1mg?

	Serial number of experiment				
	1	2	3	4	5
Dose of drug (mg)	0.3	0.4	0.6	0.8	0.9
Response to drug (mm)	54	59	60	65	70

Assume data do not follow the normal distribution.

Answer

First question: What is the aim?

Here, the aim is to "predict value from another measured variable".

Second question: What type of data it is?

These data are ratio data.

Third question: Whether the data follow the normal distribution?

Data do not follow the normal distribution (see exercise).

So, on the basis of table the most appropriate test in this condition will be "nonparametric regression".

	Type of data		
Goal	Ratio and interval data which follows normal distribution	Ratio and interval data which does not follow normal distribution and ordinal data (rank and scores)	Nominal data
Describe one group	Mean, standard deviation	Median, interquartile range	Proportion
Compare one group to a hypothetical value	One-sample *t* test	Wilcoxon test	Chi-square or binomial test
Compare two unpaired groups	Unpaired *t* test	Mann-Whitney test	Fisher's test (Chi-square for large samples)
Compare two paired groups	Paired *t* test	Wilcoxon test	McNemar's test
Compare three or more unmatched groups	One-way ANOVA	Kruskal-Wallis test	Chi-square test
Compare three or more matched groups	Repeated-measures ANOVA	Friedman test	Cochrane Q
Quantify association between two variables	Pearson correlation	Spearman correlation	Contingency coefficients
Predict value from another measured variable	Simple linear regression or nonlinear regression	Nonparametric regression	Simple logistic regression
Predict value from several measured or binomial variables	Multiple linear regression or multiple nonlinear regression		Multiple logistic regression

Example 3: 10 patients were randomly selected from psychiatry department. There anxiety scale and depression scale were measured. Data are given below:

Serial No	*Anxiety scale*	*Depression scale*
1	22	30
2	18	15
3	17	20
4	19	19
5	22	10
6	12	9
7	14	11
8	11	9
9	19	20
10	7	8

What will be the depression scale value at anxiety scale value of 15?

Answer

First question: What is the aim?

Here, the aim is to "predict value from another measured variable".

Second question: What type of data it is?

These data are ordinal data.

Third question: Whether the data follow the normal distribution?

Ordinal data do not follow the normal distribution. So, on the basis of table the most appropriate test in this condition will be "nonparametric regression".

	Type of data		
Goal	Ratio and interval data which follows normal distribution	Ratio and interval data which does not follow normal distribution and ordinal data (rank and scores)	Nominal data
Describe one group	Mean, standard deviation	Median, interquartile range	Proportion
Compare one group to a hypothetical value	One-sample *t* test	Wilcoxon test	Chi-square or binomial test
Compare two unpaired groups	Unpaired *t* test	Mann-Whitney test	Fisher's test (Chi-square for large samples)
Compare two paired groups	Paired *t* test	Wilcoxon test	McNemar's test
Compare three or more unmatched groups	One-way ANOVA	Kruskal-Wallis test	Chi-square test
Compare three or more matched groups	Repeated-measures ANOVA	Friedman test	Cochrane Q
Quantify association between two variables	Pearson correlation	Spearman correlation	Contingency coefficients
Predict value from another measured variable	Simple linear regression or nonlinear regression	Nonparametric regression	Simple logistic regression
Predict value from several measured or binomial variables	Multiple linear regression or multiple nonlinear regression		Multiple logistic regression

Example 4: A table showing the relationship between the age and signs of coronary heart disease is given below (CHD = 1, No CHD = 0). What will be the risk of occurring CHD at the age of 65 year?

Age	*CHD*	*Age*	*CHD*
22	0	40	0
23	0	41	1
24	0	46	0
27	0	47	0
28	0	48	0
30	0	49	1
30	0	49	0
32	0	50	1
33	0	51	0
35	1	51	1
38	0	52	0

Answer

First question: What is the aim?

Here, the aim is to "predict value from another measured variable".

Second question: What type of data it is?

Outcome variable is absence or presence of CHD. So, this is a nominal data. Remember that type of data should be analyzed as dependent variable.

Third question: Whether the data follow the normal distribution?

Nominal data do not follow the normal distribution so, on the basis of table the most appropriate test in this condition will be "simple logistic regression".

	Type of data		
Goal	Ratio and interval data which follows normal distribution	Ratio and interval data which does not follow normal distribution and ordinal data (rank and scores)	Nominal data
Describe one group	Mean, standard deviation	Median, interquartile range	Proportion
Compare one group to a hypothetical value	One-sample *t* test	Wilcoxon test	Chi-square or binomial test
Compare two unpaired groups	Unpaired *t* test	Mann-Whitney test	Fisher's test (Chi-square for large samples)
Compare two paired groups	Paired *t* test	Wilcoxon test	McNemar's test
Compare three or more unmatched groups	One-way ANOVA	Kruskal-Wallis test	Chi-square test
Compare three or more matched groups	Repeated-measures ANOVA	Friedman test	Cochrane Q
Quantify association between two variables	Pearson correlation	Spearman correlation	Contingency coefficients
Predict value from another measured variable	Simple linear regression or nonlinear regression	Nonparametric regression	Simple logistic regression
Predict value from several measured or binomial variables	Multiple linear regression or multiple nonlinear regression		Multiple logistic regression

PREDICT VALUE FROM SEVERAL MEASURED OR BINOMIAL VARIABLES

Here, value of one dependent variable can be predicted on the basis of more than one independent variable. Suppose you have a data set consisting of the gender, height and age of children between 5 and 10 years old. You could use multiple linear regression to predict the height of a child (dependent variable) using both age and gender as predictors (i.e. two independent variables).

Example 1: Results of a study conducted on a population are given below. Which statistical test you will use to predict the systolic blood pressure at the weight of 75 kg and serum cholesterol 170? (Assume data follow the normal distribution).

Weight	*Serum cholesterol*	*Systolic blood pressure*
51	162.2	108
52	158.0	111
56	157.0	115
56.5	155.0	116
58	154.1	117
60.1	169.1	120
59.4	181.0	124
56.1	174.9	127
61.2	180.2	122
85.5	174.0	121

Answer

First question: What is the aim?

Here, the aim is to "predict value from several measured or binomial variables".

Second question: What type of data it is?

Ratio data (cholesterol, systolic blood pressure, weight).

	Type of data		
Goal	Ratio and interval data which follows normal distribution	Ratio and interval data which does not follow normal distribution and ordinal data (rank and scores)	Nominal data
Describe one group	Mean, standard deviation	Median, interquartile range	Proportion
Compare one group to a hypothetical value	One-sample *t* test	Wilcoxon test	Chi-square or binomial test
Compare two unpaired groups	Unpaired *t* test	Mann-Whitney test	Fisher's test (Chi-square for large samples)
Compare two paired groups	Paired *t* test	Wilcoxon test	McNemar's test
Compare three or more unmatched groups	One-way ANOVA	Kruskal-Wallis test	Chi-square test
Compare three or more matched groups	Repeated-measures ANOVA	Friedman test	Cochrane Q
Quantify association between two variables	Pearson correlation	Spearman correlation	Contingency coefficients
Predict value from another measured variable	Simple linear regression or nonlinear regression	Nonparametric regression	Simple logistic regression
Predict value from several measured or binomial variables	Multiple linear regression or multiple nonlinear regression		Multiple logistic regression

Third question: Whether the data follow the normal distribution?

Data follow the normal distribution (assumed in exercise) so, on the basis of table the most appropriate test in this condition will be "multiple linear regression or multiple nonlinear regression".

Example 2: A random sample of 200 patients admitted to an adult intensive care unit (ICU) was collected to examine factors associated with death during hospital stay for ICU patients. Data was also collected on patient's age (in years), race, whether the patient had an infection at the time of ICU admission, and whether the patient had CPR administered prior to the hospital admission. Of specific interest is whether or not infection at the time of admission is associated with increased probability of death during hospital stay. Which statistical test you will use in this condition?

Answer

First question: What is the aim?

Here, the aim is to "predict value from several measured or binomial variables".

Second question: What type of data it is?

Dependent variable is death/no death which is nominal data. Independent variables are age, race, infection at the time of ICU admission, CPR administered before admission.

Third question: Whether the data follow the normal distribution?

Nominal data do not follow the normal distribution

So, on the basis of table the most appropriate test in this condition will be "multiple logistic regression regression".

	Type of data		
Goal	Ratio and interval data which follows normal distribution	Ratio and interval data which does not follow normal distribution and ordinal data (rank and scores)	Nominal data
Describe one group	Mean, standard deviation	Median, interquartile range	Proportion
Compare one group to a hypothetical value	One-sample *t* test	Wilcoxon test	Chi-square or binomial test
Compare two unpaired groups	Unpaired *t* test	Mann-Whitney test	Fisher's test (Chi-square for large samples)
Compare two paired groups	Paired *t* test	Wilcoxon test	McNemar's test
Compare three or more unmatched groups	One-way ANOVA	Kruskal-Wallis test	Chi-square test
Compare three or more matched groups	Repeated-measures ANOVA	Friedman test	Cochrane Q
Quantify association between two variables	Pearson correlation	Spearman correlation	Contingency coefficients
Predict value from another measured variable	Simple linear regression or nonlinear regression	Nonparametric regression	Simple logistic regression
Predict value from several measured or binomial variables	Multiple linear regression or multiple nonlinear regression		Multiple logistic regression

SELECTION OF STATISTICAL TEST FOR SURVIVAL TIME

Survival analysis is used for the studying the time between entry to a study and a subsequent event. Originally, the analysis was concerned with time from treatment until death, hence the name, but survival analysis is applicable to many areas in addition to mortality.

Recent examples include time to discontinuation of a contraceptive, maximum dose of bronchoconstrictor required to reduce a patient's lung function to 80% of baseline, time taken to exercise to maximum tolerance, time that a transdermal patch can be left in place, time for a leg fracture to heal.

Standard statistical techniques cannot usually be applied because the underlying distribution is rarely normal and the data are often 'censored'. A survival time is described as censored when there is a follow-up time but the event has not yet occurred or is not known to have occurred. For example, if remission time is being studied and the patient is still in remission at the end of the study, then that patient's remission time would be censored. If a patient for some reason drops out of a study before the end of the study period, then that patient's follow-up time would also be considered to be censored.

For the selection of statistical test for survival time, table is given below:

Goal	Test
Describe one group	Kaplan Meier survival curve
Compare two unpaired groups	Log-rank test or Mantel-Haenszel
Compare two paired groups	Conditional proportional hazards regression
Compare three or more unmatched groups	Cox proportional hazard regression
Compare three or more matched groups	Conditional proportional hazards regression
Quantify association between two variables	
Predict value from another measured variable	Cox proportional hazard regression
Predict value from several measured or binomial variables	Cox proportional hazard regression

For the selection of appropriate test we should know what is our goal? A test can be selected from the table according to the goal.

DESCRIBE ONE GROUP

A single group is sometime observed for time to event after an intervention.

Example: A drug rofecoxib was given to see the effect on survival of patients of colorectal cancer.

Data are given in the table below:

Treatment	*Survival time in month*
Rofecoxib	1+, 5+, 6, 6, 9+, 10, 10, 10+, 12, 12, 12, 12, 12+, 13+, 15+, 16+, 20+, 24, 24+, 27+, 32, 34+, 36+, 36+, 44+

(+ sign indicate the censored data)

Use appropriate statistical test to analyze the survival data.

Answer

Question: What is the goal?

The goal is to "describe one group" for survival analysis.

So, for the analysis of survival time in this data, most appropriate test will be "Kaplan Meier survival curve".

COMPARE TWO UNPAIRED GROUPS

Two unpaired group's survival curves are compared for any significant differences.

Example: A researcher wanted to see the effect of a new drug "N" on the mortality in the patient of a terminal disease. She recruited two groups randomly. One group was given new drug and another group was given an older established drug for the same indication, "O". Data is given in the table below. Is new drug is better as compared to old?

Treatment groups	*Survival time in months*
Drug N (N-25)	1+, 5+, 6, 6, 9+, 10, 10, 10+, 12, 12, 12, 12, 12+, 13+, 15+, 16+, 20+, 24, 24+, 27+, 32, 34+, 36+, 36+, 44+
Drug O (N-24)	3+, 6, 6, 6, 6, 8, 8, 12, 12, 12+, 15+, 16+, 18+, 18+, 20, 22+, 24, 28+, 28+, 28+, 30, 30+, 33+, 42

(+ sign indicate the censored data)

Answer

Question: What is the goal?

The goal is to "compare two unpaired groups". Here, the drug "N" and drug "O" groups are not matched. So, they are unpaired groups.

So, appropriate test will be "log-rank test or Mantel-Haenszel test".

COMPARE TWO PAIRED GROUPS

Example: In the above exercise suppose both the groups drug "N" group and drug "O" groups are matched with each other. Than what will be the appropriate test for there survival data?

Answer

Question: What is the goal?

In this condition there are two groups one of drug "N" and another of drug "O" and both are matched so now, the data is paired data not the unpaired one. So, the goal is "compared to paired group" and appropriate test will be "conditional proportional hazards regression".

COMPARE THREE OR MORE UNMATCHED GROUPS

Example: Suppose in the exercise two, there are three groups instead of two. The third group is placebo group "P". Data are given below. Which test should be used to compare survival time of all three groups?

Treatment groups	*Survival time in months*
Drug N (N-25)	1+, 5+, 6, 6, 9+, 10, 10, 10+, 12, 12, 12, 12, 12+, 13+, 15+, 16+, 20+, 24, 24+, 27+, 32, 34+, 36+, 36+, 44+
Drug O (N-24)	3+, 6, 6, 6, 6, 8, 8, 12, 12, 12+, 15+, 16+, 18+, 18+, 20, 22+, 24, 28+, 28+, 28+, 30, 30+, 33+, 42
Placebo P (N-25)	2, 5, 5, 5, 5, 7, 8, 8, 14+, 14, 16+, 20+, 24, 24, 25, 28+, 28+, 28+, 30, 30+, 33+, 42, 42, 43+,44+

(+ sign indicate the censored data)

Answer

Question: What is the goal?

The goal is "compare three or more unmatched groups".

So, the "Cox proportional hazard regression" will be the appropriate statistical test.

COMPARE THREE OR MORE MATCHED GROUPS

Example: In the exercise four, suppose all the three groups are matched with each other than what will be the appropriate test?

Answer

Question: What is the goal?

Here, as all the groups are matched so, the data is paired data. Hence, the goal will be "compare three or more matched groups".

The most appropriate test in this condition will be "conditional proportional hazards regression".

PREDICT VALUE FROM ANOTHER MEASURED VARIABLE

In this condition value of a dependent variable can be predicted on the basis of another independent variable.

Example: Survival outcomes of two treatments (treatment 1 and treatment 2) are given below. If you want to see the effect of age on survival time, which statistical test you will use?

Patients number	*Survival days*	*Outcome*	*Treatment*	*Age*
1	1	Died	2	75
2	1	Died	2	79
3	4	Died	2	85
4	5	Died	2	76
5	6	Unknown	2	66
6	8	Died	1	75
7	9	Survived	2	72
8	9	Died	2	70
9	12	Died	1	71
10	15	Unknown	1	73
11	22	Died	2	66
12	25	Survived	1	73
13	37	Died	1	68
14	55	Died	1	59
15	72	Survived	1	61

Answer

Question: What is the goal?

The goal is "predict value from another measured variable".

So, the "Cox proportional hazard regression" will be the appropriate statistical test.

PREDICT VALUE FROM SEVERAL MEASURED OR BINOMIAL VARIABLES

Here, again value of dependent variable can be predicted on the basis of independent variables. The prediction is not done on the basis of just one independent variable, but many independent variables.

Example: In the exercise six, suppose one more variable is added, i.e. sex (1—male, 2— female), and now we want to predict the dependent variable (survival time) on the basis of two independent variable age and sex than what will be the most appropriate statistical test?

Patients number	*Survival days*	*Outcome*	*Treatment*	*Age*	*Sex*
1	1	Died	2	75	1
2	1	Died	2	79	2
3	4	Died	2	85	2
4	5	Died	2	76	1
5	6	Unknown	2	66	2
6	8	Died	1	75	2
7	9	Survived	2	72	1
8	9	Died	2	70	1
9	12	Died	1	71	1
10	15	Unknown	1	73	2
11	22	Died	2	66	1
12	25	Survived	1	73	1
13	37	Died	1	68	1
14	55	Died	1	59	2
15	72	Survived	1	61	1

Answer

Question: What is the goal?

Here, prediction will be done on the basis of two independent variables (age and sex), so goal is "predict value from several measured or binomial variables".

So, the appropriate test in this condition will be "Cox proportional hazard regression".

Chapter 5

One-tailed or Two-tailed

Statistical tests can be calculated as one-tailed or two-tailed. Before starting the research a researcher has some hypothesis. On the basis of hypothesis she designs the research protocol. Suppose she wants to see the effect of a new antihypertensive drug, then she may have one of the two hypotheses. One, new antihypertensive drug will always decrease the blood pressure and second, this new drug may decrease the blood pressure or may increase the blood pressure. In the former condition, one-tailed test should be used and in later condition two-tailed test should be used. But the question is how she is so much sure that it will always decrease the blood pressure? This new drug may decrease the blood pressure or may increase the same. One-tailed test should only be used when the hypothesis is based on strong scientific research. It should be used when researcher is sure that either there will be no effect of intervention or the effect will be in one direction. If there is any confusion it is better to use two-tailed test. In medical research we should always use the two-tailed test so that, any effect observed even in opposite direction can be exploited for further research.

Before using the table for various tests we should first confirm whether this table is for one-tailed or two-tailed tests? Sometimes only one-tailed or two-tailed table is given. We can see the value of two-tailed test in one-tailed table and vice versa by using this conversion table.

Table you have	*Operation*	*To get ...*
One-tailed	Divide P by 2	Two-tailed test for $P/2$
Two-tailed	Multiply P by 2	One-tailed test for $2P$

CHAPTER 6

Test for Homogeneity of Variances

Applying the statistical test like unpaired *t* test or one-way ANOVA involves some assumptions about the data. These are as follows:

1. Study subjects should be selected randomly.
2. Variables of the study should be distributed normally.
3. There should be homogeneity of variances between the study groups.

These assumptions should be verified before applying the tests.

The meaning of homogeneity of variances is that variances of all the groups in the study are almost same. There are various specific tests for checking the homogeneity of variances. Tests for checking homogeneity of variances are:

1. Variance ratio test
2. "F" max test
3. Bartlett's test
4. Cochran's test
5. Scheffe's test

If we are using the software for analysis than all the tests for homogeneity can be performed easily. Here, we will understand simplest one "variance ratio test".

VARIANCE RATIO TEST

It is the ratio of maximum variance to minimum variance. Suppose, we are having two study groups, group A and group B. The standard deviation of group A is SA and group B is SB than the variance of group A will be SA^2 and variance of group B will be SB^2. If variance of group B is larger than group A ($SB^2 > SA^2$) than variance ratio will be $F = SB^2/SA^2$.

The significance of F can be seen in F table. The degree of freedom is $n_a - 1$ and $n_b - 1$ (n_a : No. of subjects in group A, n_b : No. of subjects in group B). F table gives variance ratio at different significance level with the help of degree of freedoms of two samples. When study groups are more than two, then ratio should be taken of largest variance to smallest variance. If, F-value (variance ratio) is greater than value obtained in the table at 5% of significance, it can be said that variance of two groups are different significantly and homogeneity of variance is not there.

Example: The variances observed in clotting time of plasma with two treatments are given. Can we conclude that there is homogeneity of variances?

	Group A	*Group B*
Sample size	9	9
Variance (SD^2)	1.21	0.12

Variance ratio (F) = Largest variance/smallest variance
= 1.21/0.12
= 10.08

Degree of freedom for group A = $n_a - 1 = 9 - 1 = 8$

Degree of freedom for group B = $n_b - 1 = 9 - 1 = 8$

At this degree of freedom from both the groups value in the F table at the significance of 0.5% is 7.50. The value of variance ratio (F) is more than this value so, we can conclude that there is no homogeneity of variances between the two groups.

CHAPTER 7

Post-hoc Tests of ANOVA

ANOVA calculation tests the null hypothesis that all the study groups are sampled from the distribution which has same mean. A significant ANOVA test indicates that study group's means are not equal and largest and smallest means are significantly different but it will not tell about the comparison of other groups. Suppose we were interested in testing a new intervention for a particular disease and we recruited three groups randomly. First group was given new drug, second group was given older established drug and third group was given placebo. One-way ANOVA was significant. It means all the three study groups are not from same population, there mean is significantly different. Suppose highest mean is of placebo group and lowest mean is of established drug group so, we can say that there is a significant difference between placebo and established drug group but what about placebo and new drug group comparison or new drug and old drug group comparison? Various types of comparison within the group can be done by the some tests and they are called "post-hoc tests". Other terminologies with slightly different meanings are also used like "post-tests" or "multiple comparison tests" or "planned comparison tests" and "orthogonal comparison tests". Post-hoc tests should be performed only when ANOVA is significant.

There are various types of post-hoc tests are available and they can be performed easily by the software like SPSS. At our level, we require the knowledge of only few important post-hoc tests.

Post-hoc tests available are as follow:

A. *When equal variance is assumed*

1. LSD (Least Significant Difference) test
2. Bonferroni test
3. Sidak test
4. Scheffe's test

5. Ryan-Einot-Gabriel-Welsch F test
6. Ryan-Einot-Gabriel-Welsch range test
7. Student-Newman-Keuls test
8. Tukey's (Honest Significant Difference, HSD) test
9. Tukey's-*b* test
10. Duncan test
11. Hochberg's GT2 test
12. Gabriel test
13. Waller-Duncan test
14. Dunnett's test

B. *Equal variance is not assumed*

1. Tamhane's T2 test
2. Dunnett's T3 test
3. Games-Howell test
4. Dunnett's C test

We will deal with few important tests only. These few tests are sufficient for most of the research questions.

1. *LSD (Least Significant Difference) test:* This is equivalent to running a *t* test. Alpha level (type 1 error) is not controlled. This test is most sensitive but least specific as alpha level is not controlled. Since, it is unlikely to miss a difference that is real, it is most powerful test but it is also least conservative test as it is more prone to commit alpha error.
2. *Bonferroni test:* To compare all possible pair of means alpha level is corrected by dividing the alpha value by possible pairs of mean. Suppose there are three study groups. So comparison will be between these three means. So there will be three pairs of mean. Hence, corrected alpha will be = alpha/3.
3. *Sidak test:* To compare all possible pair of means. Sidak test is slightly more powerful as compared to Bonferroni test alpha 0.05 But equivalent at 0.01.Alpha level is corrected.

4. *Scheffe's test:* To compare all possible pairs and all possible combinations of means. Alpha is corrected. Corrected alpha = alpha/no. of all possible pairs and combinations.

   Scheffe's procedure is perhaps the most popular of the post hoc procedures, the most flexible, and the most conservative (highly specific).

   Scheffe's procedure corrects alpha for all pairwise or simple comparisons of means, but also for all complex comparisons of means as well. Complex comparisons involve contrasts of more than two means at a time. As a result, Scheffe's is also the least statistically powerful procedure. Forsythe's post hoc procedure is a modification of the Scheffe test for situations with heterogeneity of variance.
5. *Student-Newman-Keuls test:* This is a stepwise test for ordered means where the alpha level depends upon the number of "steps apart" each of the means are from each other.

   It does not provides sufficient protection against alpha slippage and should probably be avoided.
6. *Tukey's (Honest Significant Difference, HSD) test:* For all possible pairwise comparison. Sample sizes must be equal but a revised version permits unequal sample sizes (i.e. Tukey-Kramer) alpha corrected.
7. *Duncan test:* Multiple range test. This is a stepwise test for ordered means.
8. *Dunnett's test:* It compares a control group with all other groups.

   Except Duncan test all other test are also pairwise test.

WHICH POST-HOC TEST YOU WILL SELECT FOR YOUR RESEARCH?

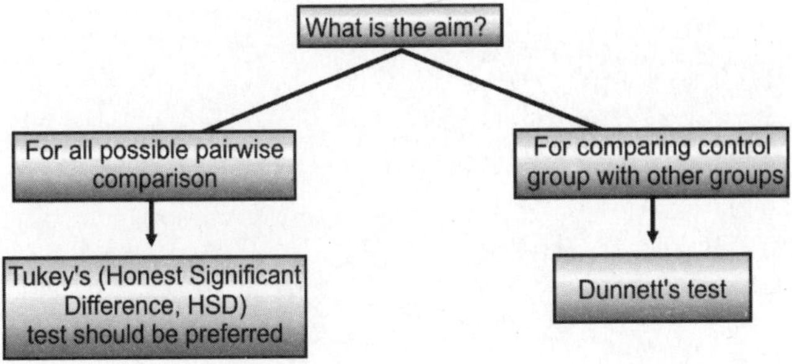

CHAPTER 8

Bonus Reading

CHECK LIST FOR THE APPRAISAL OF STATISTICAL ASPECTS OF THE RESEARCH PAPER

1. *Have the authors set the scene correctly?*
   a. Have they determined whether their groups are comparable and, if necessary adjusted for baseline differences?
   b. What sort of data they got and have they used appropriate statistical tests?
   c. If statistical tests in the paper are obscure why have the author chosen to use them?
   d. Have the data been analyzed according to original study protocol?
2. *Paired data, tails and outliers:*
   a. Were paired test performed on paired data?
   b. Was a two-tailed performed whenever the effect of an intervention could conveivably be a negative one?
   c. Were outliers analyzed with both common sense and appropriate statistical adjustments?
3. *Correlation, regression and causation:*
   a. Has correlation been distinguished from regression and has the correlation coefficient (r-value) been calculated and interpreted correctly?
   b. Have assumptions been made about the nature and directions of causality?
4. *Probability and confidence:*
   a. Have P-value been calculated and interpreted appropriately?
   b. Have confidence interval calculated and do the author's conclusions reflect them?
5. *Have authors expressed their results in terms of the likely harm or benefit that an individual patient can expect, such as:*
   a. Relative risk reduction

b. Absolute risk reduction
c. Number needed to treat
d. Odd ratio

(Greenhalgh T. How to Read a Paper? BMJ 1997;315:93).

COMMON PITFALLS RELATED TO STATISTICAL ERRORS IN MEDICAL RESEARCH

Statistical Errors and Deficiencies Related to the Design of a Study

1. Study aims and primary outcome measures not clearly stated or unclear.
2. Failure to report number of participants or observations (sample size).
3. Failure to report withdrawals from the study.
4. No apriori sample size calculation/effect size estimation (power calculation).
5. No clear apriori statement or description of the null hypothesis under investigation.
6. Failure to use and report randomization.
7. Method of randomization not clearly stated.
8. Failure to use and report blinding if possible.
9. Failure to report initial equality of baseline characteristics and comparability of study groups.
10. Use of an inappropriate control group.
11. Inappropriate testing for equality of baseline characteristics.

Statistical Errors and Deficiencies Related to Data Analysis

1. Use of wrong statistical tests:
   - Incompatibility of statistical test with type of data examined

- Unpaired tests for paired data or vice versa
- Inappropriate use of parametric methods
- Use of an inappropriate test for the hypothesis under investigation

2. Inflation of type I error
   - Failure to include a multiple comparison correction
   - Inappropriate post-hoc subgroup analysis
3. Typical errors with student's *t*-test
   - Failure to prove test assumptions
   - Unequal sample sizes for paired *t*-test
   - Improper multiple pairwise comparisons of more than two groups
   - Use of an unpaired *t*-test for paired data or vice versa
4. Typical errors with Chi-square tests:
   - No Yates-continuity correction reported if small numbers
   - Use of Chi-square when expected numbers in a cell are < 5
   - No explicit statement of the tested null hypotheses
5. Failure to use multivariety techniques to adjust for confounding factors.

Errors Related to the Documentation of Statistical Methods Applied

1. Failure to specify/define all tests used clear and correctly:
   - Failure to state number of tails
   - Failure to state if test was paired or unpaired
2. Wrong names for statistical tests.
3. Referring to unusual or obscure methods without explanation or reference.
4. Failure to specify which test was applied on a given set of data if more than one test was done.

Statistical Errors and Deficiencies Related to the Presentation of Study Data

1. Inadequate graphical or numerical description of basic data:
   - Mean but no indication of variability of the data.
   - Giving statistical error instead of standard deviation to describe data
   - Use of mean (standard deviation) to describe non-normal data
   - Failure to define ± notion for describing variability or use of unlabeled error bars
2. Inappropriate and poor reporting of results:
   - Results given only as P-values, no confidence intervals given
   - Confidence intervals given for each group rather than for contrasts
   - "P = NS", "P < 0.05" or other arbitrary thresholds instead of reporting exact P-values
   - Numerical information given to an unrealistic level of precision

Statistical Errors and Deficiencies Related to the Interpretation of Study Findings

1. Wrong interpretation of results:
   - "Nonsignificant" interpreted as "no effect",or "no difference"
   - Drawing conclusions not supported by the study data.
   - Significance claimed without data analysis or statistical test mentioned
2. Poor interpretation of results:
   - Disregard for type II error when reporting non-significant results
   - Missing discussion of the problem of multiple significance testing if done
   - Failure to discuss sources of potential bias and confounding factors

CHAPTER 9

Solved Exercises

Exercise 1: In the patients undergoing surgery for perforated eye injuries maintenance of intraocular pressure is very important. A raised intraocular pressure may have deleterious effects on eye. Metoclopramide is a prokinetic drug which is given to hasten the gastric emptying in emergency surgeries including eye surgeries. In this study aim of the researchers is to see the effect of metoclopramide on intraocular pressure and also on change in intraocular pressure after administration of muscle relaxant succinlycholine and tracheal intubation. Researcher divided 60 patients who came for elective eye surgery into two groups of 30 each by random table. Group C was given 2 ml of saline and group M was given 2 ml of metoclopramide 30 minutes before induction of anesthesia by thiopentone. Intraocular pressure measured in both the eye pre-and post-drug treatment and at succinylcholine and tracheal intubation. Table of findings are given below. Which statistical test should be used to compare the two groups and also to see the effect of tracheal intubation and succinylcholine administration on intraocular pressure?

(Sudheera KS, Bhardwaj M, Yaddanapudi S. Effect of Intravenous Metoclopramide on Intraocular Pressure: A Prospective, Randomized, Double Blind, Placebo Controlled Study. J Postgrad Med 2008; 54:195-8).

Time	*Group C (N-30)*	*Group M (N-30)*
Baseline	11.8 ± 1.5	11.9 ± 1.5
2 min after drug test	11.7 ± 1.5	11.1 ± 1.5
5 min after drug test	11.0 ± 1.5	10.9 ± 1.3
15 min after drug test	11.0 ± 1.3	10.9 ± 0.9
Before thiopentone	11.2 ± 1.1	11.0 ± 1.2
After thiopentone	7.0 ± 1.8	6.6 ± 1.4
2 min after intubation	16.3 ± 2.1	15.6 ± 2.4
5 min after intubation	13.4 ± 1.9	12.8 ± 2.3

(All values are expressed in mean ± standard deviation)

You are supposed to compare two set of data for different aims. To see the effect of metoclopramide on intraocular pressure, drug and placebo group should be compared and to see the effect of tracheal intubation and succinylcholine administration on intraocular pressure. All the paired data need to be compared. Distribution of data checked and found to be distributed normally.

Exercise 2: The optimal target range for blood glucose in critically ill patients is not clear. Researchers were interested in knowing the effect of tight sugar control on the mortality of critically ill patients. For that they randomly divided critically ill patients of intensive care unit into two groups. Group A was assigned to tight blood sugar control (81 to 108 mg per deciliter) and group B was assigned to conventional target (180 mg or less per deciliter). Primary endpoint was death from any cause within 90 days of randomization. Data for death is given below. Which test of significance should be used to see the difference between two groups?

(The NICE-SUGAR Study Investigators. Intensive versus Conventional Glucose Control in Critically Ill Patients. N Engl J Med 2009; 360:1283-97).

Outcome	*Group A (Intensive glucose control)*	*Group B (Conventional control)*
No. of death up to 90 days	829/3010	751/3012

Exercise 3: Researchers decided to estimate the hepatoprotective effects of the methanolic seed extract of Eugenia jambolana Lam. They decided to carry an animal study. For that they used the rats. The rats were divided into six groups, each group consisting of six rats. Hepatotoxicity produced by the ccl_4.

1st group—control received by subcutaneous administration of liquid paraffin only 1 ml/kg on alternate days, for one week.

2nd group—carbon tetrachloride (CCl_4) subcutaneously, in a suspension of liquid paraffin (1:2 v/v), at a dose of 1 ml/kg body weight, on alternate days, for a week.

3rd group—positive control by Liver-52 orally daily and carbon tetrachloride (CCl_4), in a suspension of liquid paraffin (1:2 v/v), at a dose of 1 ml/kg body weight, on alternate days, for a week, subcutaneously.

4th group—orally administered the extract of Eugenia jambolana Lam (100 mg/kg) daily and carbon tetrachloride (CCl_4), in a suspension of liquid paraffin (1:2 v/v) at a dose of 1 ml/kg body weight, on alternate days, for a week, by the subcutaneous route.

5th group—orally administered the extract of Eugenia jambolana Lam (200 mg/kg) daily and carbon tetrachloride (CCl_4), in a suspension of liquid paraffin (1:2 v/v) at a dose of 1 ml/kg body weight, on alternate days, for a week, by the subcutaneous route.

6th group—orally administered the extract of Eugenia jambolana Lam. (400 mg/kg) daily and carbon tetrachloride (CCl_4), in a suspension of liquid paraffin (1:2 v/v) at a dose of 1 ml/kg body weight, on alternate days, for a week, by the subcutaneous route.

On the eighth day, the animals were sacrificed by decapitation. Through an incision made on the jugular vein, blood was collected. The blood and serum were separated by centrifugation and used for estimation of biochemical parameters that is glutamate oxaloacetate transaminase (GOT), glutamate pyruvate transaminase (GPT), alkaline phosphatase (ALP) and acid phosphatase (ACP).

Which statistical test you will use to analyze the data of this study? Data table is given below. (Data follow normal distribution).

(Sisodia SS, Bhatnagar M. Hepatoprotective Activity of Eugenia jambolana Lam in Carbon Tetrachloride treated Rats. Indian J Pharmacol 2009;41:23-7).

Group/ treatment	*GOT U/L*	*GPT U/L*	*ALP K A Units*	*ACP K A Units*
Group I Control with LP	37.78 ± 7.26	46.69 ± 10.74	12.45 ± 2.99	6.51 ± 0.52
Group II LP + CCl_4	93.16 ± 7.92	99.68 ± 11.10	58.84 ± 14.75	14.01 ± 2.48
Group III LP + CCl_4 + Liv.52® (1 ml/kg)	52.14 ± 3.14	55.95 ± 5.57	27.79 ± 3.99	9.33 ± 0.98
Group IV LP + CCl_4 + MT (100 mg/kg)	75.11 ± 3.57	78.66 ± 4.87	54.71 ± 3.49	11.92 ± 0.49
Group V LP + CCl_4 + MT (200 mg/kg)	51.50 ± 2.08	73.94 ± 3.82	43.61 ± 5.54	10.71 ± 0.80
Group VI LP + CCl_4 + MT (400 mg/kg)	53.28 ± 6.97	68.50 ± 4.11	40.46 ± 3.05	10.72 ± 1.03

(Values are represented as mean ± SEM (n = 6) in each group)

Exercise 4: Femoral head preserving core decompression and bone grafting have shown excellent result in preventing collapse. The use of vascularized grafts has shown better clinical results. The vascular pedicle bone graft is easy to perform operation and does not require special equipment. Researcher analyzed and reports a series of patients of osteonecrosis of femoral head treated by core decompression and vascular pedicle grafting of part of iliac crest based on deep circumflex iliac vessels. He did the retrospective study of 31 patients of osteonecrosis of femoral head in stage II and III treated with core decompression and vascular pedicle grafting by using part of iliac crest with deep circumflex iliac vessels. He compared pre and post surgery outcomes by Harris hip score. Which test you will select to analyze the effect of surgery on Harris hip score? Data is given below.

(Babhulkar S. Osteonecrosis of Femoral Head: Treatment by Core Decompression and Vascular Pedicle Grafting. Indian J Orthop 2009;43:27-35).

Serial No.	*Preoperative score*	*Postoperative score*
1	49	56
2	57	48
3	57	57
4	48	50
5	48	55
6	47	48
7	50	49
8	48	56
9	55	48
10	50	50
11	67	55
12	50	49
13	65	57
14	49	57
15	56	48
16	48	48
17	50	47

(Contd.)

(Contd.)

18	56	50
19	49	48
20	57	55
21	56	50
22	48	67
23	57	50
24	50	65
25	55	49
26	48	56
27	49	48
28	56	50
29	48	56
30	50	49
31	55	57

Exercise 5: Smoking in the pregnancy associated with adverse fetal outcome. Researcher wants to compare pregnancy outcomes between women who stopped smoking in early pregnancy and those who either did not smoke in pregnancy or continued to smoke. For this they did prospective cohort study. 2504 nulliparous women who were participating in the screening for pregnancy endpoints (SCOPE) study were grouped by maternal smoking status at 15 (± 1) week's gestation. Main outcome measures were spontaneous preterm birth and small for gestational age infants (birth weight < 10th customized centile). They wanted to compare odds of these outcomes between stopped smokers and nonsmokers, and between current smokers and stopped smokers and to adjust the results for demographic and clinical risk factors. Which statistical test should be selected to analyze this data?

(Lesley M E, Gustaaf A, Eliza C, Stewart A, Chappell S, Hunter M, et al. Spontaneous Preterm Birth and Small for Gestational Age Infants in Women Who Stop Smoking Early in Pregnancy: Prospective Cohort Study. BMJ 2009;338:1081).

	Nonsmoker (n-1992)	*Stopped smoking (n-261)*	*Current smoker (n-251)*
Spontaneous preterm birth	88	10	25
Small for gestational age	195	27	42

Exercise 6: Previous studies have demonstrated a strong association of hypertension and renal disease with gout. Nevertheless, controversy remains concerning serum uric acid concentration as an independent factor of hypertension. Researchers decided to explore the relationship between systolic blood pressure (SBP) and diastolic blood pressure (DBP) with serum uric acid levels through an observational study. A total of 5,564 subjects recruited in the study. There systolic and diastolic blood pressure and serum uric acid level measured. Which statistical test you will use to estimate the association between blood pressure and uric acid concentration in blood? (Assume normal distribution).

(Ouppatham S, Bancha S, Choovichian P. The Relationship of Hyperuricemia and Blood Pressure in the Thai Army Population. J Postgrad Med 2008;54:259-62).

Mean SBP (mm Hg)	*Mean DBP (mm Hg)*	*Mean concentration of uric acid in serum(mg/dl)*
128.73 ± 17.06	81.62 ± 11	6.54 ± 1.71

(All values are expressed in mean ± SD)

Exercise 7: Researcher decided to determine whether early initiated anti-inflammatory therapy with prolonged high dose inhaled glucocorticoids influences the occurrence and severity of recurrent wheeze after respiratory syncytial virus related lower respiratory tract infections. They did a randomized double blind placebo controlled trial for this at pediatric departments of 19 Dutch clinical centers. Participants were 243 previously, healthy infants (126 boys, 117 girls) aged less than 13 months and admitted to hospital with respiratory syncytial virus infection. 119 were randomized to receive beclomethasone and 124 to receive placebo. 200 µg extra fine hydrofluoroalkane (HFA) beclomethasone dipropionate twice daily or matched placebo administered by a pressurized metered dose inhaler and a spacer during the first three months after hospital admission. The primary outcome was the number of days with wheeze in the year after the three months intervention period. Select the appropriate statistical test to compare drug and placebo.

(Marieke J J , Maroeska M , Job B l, Jan L L , Louis J , on behalf of the RSV Corticosteroid Study Group. The Effect of High Dose Inhaled Corticosteroids on Wheeze in Infants after Respiratory Syncytial Virus Infection: Randomized Double Blind Placebo Controlled Trial. BMJ 2009;338:b897).

	Beclomethasone group (n-119)	*Placebo group (n-124)*
No. of days of wheezing	1761/33568	2301/36556

Exercise 8: Surgical ventricular reconstruction is a specific procedure designed to reduce left ventricular volume in patients with heart failure caused by coronary artery disease. Researchers conducted a trial to address the question of whether surgical ventricular reconstruction

added to coronary artery bypass grafting (CABG) would decrease the rate of death or hospitalization for cardiac causes, as compared with CABG alone. Between September 2002 and January 2006, a total of 1000 patients with an ejection fraction of 35% or less, coronary artery disease that was amenable to CABG, and dominant anterior left ventricular dysfunction that was amenable to surgical ventricular reconstruction were randomly assigned to undergo either CABG alone (499 patients) or CABG with surgical ventricular reconstruction (501 patients). The primary outcome was a composite of death from any cause and hospitalization for cardiac causes. The median follow-up was 48 months. Researcher wants to compare both the groups by survival time (cumulative event rates from the time of randomization). Which is the most appropriate test for this condition?

(Jones, Robert H, Velazquez, Eric J, Michler, Robert E, et al. Coronary Bypass Surgery with or without Surgical Ventricular Reconstruction. N Engl J Med 2009:29).

Exercise 9: Researchers were interested in knowing the effect of extract of an ayurvedic herb "Tinospora cordifolia". They decided to assess the efficacy of Tinospora cordifolia extract (TCE) in HIV positive patients in randomized double blind placebo controlled trial. 68 HIV positive participants were randomly assigned to two groups to receive either TCE or placebo for six months. After clinical examination TLC, DLC, ESR, platelet count, hemoglobin and CD4 count were done. The hematological investigations were repeated at bimonthly intervals and CD4 count was repeated at the end of the study. Select the appropriate statistical test to see the difference between herb and placebo. (Data do not follow the normal distribution).

(Kalikar MV, Thawani VR, Varadpande UK, Sontakke SD, Singh RP, Khiyani RK. Immunomodulatory Effect of Tinospora Cordifolia Extract in Human Immuno Deficiency Virus Positive Patients. Indian J Pharmacol 2008;40:107-10).

	Tinospora cordifolia	*Placebo*
CD4	296.2 ± 195.2	268.0 ± 205.3
TLC	5647.3 ± 1715.0	5433.8 ± 1766.1
Neutrophils	60.6 ± 8.9	58.1 ± 10.1
Lymphocytes	32.7 ± 8.9	32.6 ± 6.9
Eosinophils	3.5 ± 1.2	3.1 ± 1.4
Monocytes	3.8 ± 1.5	3.2 ± 1.2
ESR	17.3 ± 5.1	19.1 ± 7.7
Platelets	2.0 ± 0.4	2.0 ± 0.5
Hemoglobin	11.8 ± 1.36	11.7 ± 1.6

ANSWERS

Exercise 1

Here you are supposed to compare two set of data for different aims. To see the effect of metoclopramide on intraocular pressure, drug and placebo, groups should be compared and to see the effect of tracheal intubation and succinylcholine administration on intraocular pressure all the paired data need to be compared. Distribution of data checked and found to be distributed normally.

First test

First question: What is the aim?

Here, the aim is to "compare two unpaired groups".

Second question: What type of data it is?

Intraocular pressure fulfill the all criteria of ratio data.

Third question: Whether the data follow the normal distribution?

Yes, data follow the normal distribution:

So, after looking at the table we can say that "Unpaired *t* test" is appropriate test for this aim.

Second test

First question: What is the aim?

Here, the aim is to "compare three or more matched groups".

Second question: What type of data it is?

Intraocular pressure fulfill the all criteria of ratio data.

Third question: Whether the data follow the normal distribution?

Yes, data follow the normal distribution.

So, appropriate test in this condition will be the "Repeated-measures ANOVA". As we had already discussed that ANOVA only tell about the difference in mean between the groups it does not tell which group is better. In this condition you will use post-hoc tests of ANOVA. So if you want to compare all pair of means than Tukey's HSD test is better and if you want to compare other means with control only then Dunnett's test is better post-hoc test.

	Type of data		
Goal	Ratio and interval data which follows normal distribution	Ratio and interval data which does not follow normal distribution and ordinal data (rank and scores)	Nominal data
Describe one group	Mean, standard deviation	Median, interquartile range	Proportion

(*Contd.*)

(*Contd.*)

	Type of data		
Compare one group to a hypothetical value	One-sample *t* test	Wilcoxon test	Chi-square or binomial test
Compare two unpaired groups	Unpaired *t* test	Mann-Whitney test	Fisher's test (Chi-square for large samples)
Compare two paired groups	Paired *t* test	Wilcoxon test	McNemar's test
Compare three or more unmatched groups	One-way ANOVA	Kruskal-Wallis test	Chi-square test
Compare three or more matched groups	Repeated-measures ANOVA	Friedman test	Cochrane Q
Quantify association between two variables	Pearson correlation	Spearman correlation	Contingency coefficients
Predict value from another measured variable	Simple linear regression or nonlinear regression	Nonparametric regression	Simple logistic regression
Predict value from several measured or binomial variables	Multiple linear regression or multiple nonlinear regression		Multiple logistic regression

Exercise 2

In this study researcher wants to see the effect of tight sugar control on mortality within 90 days.

First question: What is the aim?

Here, the aim is "compare two unpaired groups".

Second question: What type of data it is?

Death/survival fulfill the all criteria of nominal data.

Third question: Whether the data follow the normal distribution?

Nominal data do not follow the normal distribution.

Here, the sample size is large so both Fisher's test and Chi-square test can be used.

	Type of data		
Goal	Ratio and interval data which follows normal distribution	Ratio and interval data which does not follow normal distribution and ordinal data (rank and scores)	Nominal data
Describe one group	Mean, SD	Median, interquartile range	Proportion
Compare one group to a hypothetical value	One-sample *t* test	Wilcoxon test	Chi-square or binomial test
Compare two unpaired groups	Unpaired *t* test	Mann-Whitney test	Fisher's test (Chi-square for large samples)
Compare two paired groups	Paired *t* test	Wilcoxon test	McNemar's test
Compare three or more unmatched groups	One-way ANOVA	Kruskal-Wallis test	Chi-square test

(*Contd.*)

(*Contd.*)

	Type of data		
Compare three or more matched groups	Repeated-measures ANOVA	Friedman test	Cochrane Q
Quantify association between two variables	Pearson correlation	Spearman correlation	Contingency coefficients
Predict value from another measured variable	Simple linear regression or nonlinear regression	Nonparametric regression	Simple logistic regression
Predict value from several measured or binomial variables	Multiple linear regression or multiple nonlinear regression		Multiple logistic regression

Exercise 3

In this study researchers wanted to see the effect of a herb (Eugenia jambolana Lam) on ccl_4 induced hepatotoxicity.

First question: What is the aim?

Here, the aim is "compare three or more unmatched groups".

Second question: What type of data it is?

All the parameters are ratio data.

Third question: Whether the data follow the normal distribution?

It is given in the exercise that data follow the normal distribution.

So if we look at the table, ideal test in this condition will be "one-way ANOVA". As we know that post-hoc test of ANOVA should be performed after ANOVA for within group comparison. If we want to compare all pairs of means with each other than *Tukey's HSD test or LSD* (prefer tukeys) should be performed and for comparison of all means with control *Dunnett's test* should be performed.

	Type of data		
Goal	Ratio and interval data which follows normal distribution	Ratio and interval data which does not follow normal distribution and ordinal data (rank and scores)	Nominal data
Describe one group	Mean, SD	Median, interquartile range	Proportion
Compare one group to a hypothetical value	One-sample *t* test	Wilcoxon test	Chi-square or binomial test
Compare two unpaired groups	Unpaired *t* test	Mann-Whitney test	Fisher's test (Chi-square for large samples)
Compare two paired groups	Paired *t* test	Wilcoxon test	McNemar's test
Compare three or more unmatched groups	One-way ANOVA	Kruskal-Wallis test	Chi-square test
Compare three or more matched groups	Repeated-measures ANOVA	Friedman test	Cochrane Q

(*Contd.*)

(*Contd.*)

	Type of data		
Quantify association between two variables	Pearson correlation	Spearman correlation	Contingency coefficients
Predict value from another measured variable	Simple linear regression or nonlinear regression	Nonparametric regression	Simple logistic regression
Predict value from several measured or binomial variables	multiple linear regression or Multiple nonlinear regression		Multiple logistic regression

Exercise 4

In this condition author wants to see the effect of surgical technique on Morris hip score.

First question: What is the aim?

Here, the aim is "compare two paired groups". Pre- and postinterventional studies are paired data.

Second question: What type of data it is?

As we know, rank and scores are ordinal data. So, Morris hip score is an ordinal data.

Third question: Whether the data follow the normal distribution?

Ordinal data do not follow the normal distribution.

So, on the basis of table, the most appropriate test in this condition will be "Wilcoxon test" (Wilcoxon signed rank test) and it should be two-tailed.

	Type of data		
Goal	Ratio and interval data which follows normal distribution	Ratio and interval data which does not follow normal distribution and ordinal data (rank and scores)	Nominal data
Describe one group	Mean, standard deviation	Median, interquartile range	Proportion
Compare one group to a hypothetical value	One-sample *t* test	Wilcoxon test	Chi-square or binomial test
Compare two unpaired groups	Unpaired *t* test	Mann-Whitney test	Fisher's test (Chi-square for large samples)
Compare two paired groups	Paired *t* test	Wilcoxon test	McNemar's test
Compare three or more unmatched groups	One-way ANOVA	Kruskal-Wallis test	Chi-square test
Compare three or more matched groups	Repeated-measures ANOVA	Friedman test	Cochrane Q
Quantify association between two variables	Pearson correlation	Spearman correlation	Contingency coefficients
Predict value from another measured variable	Simple linear regression or nonlinear regression	Nonparametric regression	Simple logistic regression

(*Contd.*)

(Contd.)

	Type of data	
Predict value from several measured or binomial variables	Multiple linear regression or multiple nonlinear regression	Multiple logistic regression

Exercise 5

Here, researcher not only wants to compare odds of outcome between the groups but also wants to adjust that outcome for demographical and clinical risk factor.

First question: What is the aim?

Here, the aim is "predict value from several measured or binomial variables" . Researcher wants to predict the odds of outcome with the variables (demographic and clinical risk factors).

Second question: What type of data it is?

The number of preterm infant and small for gestational age is nominal data. We can count but cannot measure.

Third question: Whether the data follow the normal distribution?

Nominal data do not follow the normal distribution.

So, on the basis of table, the most appropriate test in this condition will be "multiple logistic regression".

Simple comparison without the adjustment could have been done by the Fisher's test or Chi-square test.

	Type of data		
Goal	Ratio and interval data which follows normal distribution	Ratio and interval data which does not follow normal distribution and ordinal data (rank and scores)	Nominal data
Describe one group	Mean, standard deviation	Median, interquartile range	Proportion
Compare one group to a hypothetical value	One-sample *t* test	Wilcoxon test	Chi-square or binomial test
Compare two unpaired groups	Unpaired *t* test	Mann-Whitney test	Fisher's test (Chi-square for large samples)
Compare two paired groups	Paired *t* test	Wilcoxon test	McNemar's test
Compare three or more unmatched groups	One-way ANOVA	Kruskal-Wallis test	Chi-square test
Compare three or more matched groups	Repeated-measures ANOVA	Friedman test	Cochrane Q
Quantify association between two variables	Pearson correlation	Spearman correlation	Contingency coefficients
Predict value from another measured variable	Simple linear regression or nonlinear regression	Nonparametric regression	Simple logistic regression

(Contd.)

(*Contd.*)

	Type of data		
Predict value from several measured or binomial variables	Multiple linear regression or multiple nonlinear regression		Multiple logistic regression

Exercise 6

The aim of researchers is to measure the association between SBP, DBP and serum uric acid concentration.

First question: What is the aim?

Here the aim is "quantify association between two variables". So, first pair of two variables is SBP and serum uric acid concentration and second pair is DBP and serum uric acid concentration.

Second question: What type of data it is?

The data is ratio data.

Third question: Whether the data follow the normal distribution?

We assume they follow the normal distribution.

So, on the basis of table, the most appropriate test in this condition will be "Pearson correlation" (between SBP and uric acid concentration and DBP and uric acid concentration in serum).

	Type of data		
Goal	Ratio and interval data which follows normal distribution	Ratio and interval data which does not follow normal distribution and ordinal data (rank and scores)	Nominal data

(*Contd.*)

(*Contd.*)

	Type of data		
Describe one group	Mean, standard deviation	Median, interquartile range	Proportion
Compare one group to a hypothetical value	One-sample *t* test	Wilcoxon test	Chi-square or binomial test
Compare two unpaired groups	Unpaired *t* test	Mann-Whitney test	Fisher's test (Chi-square for large samples)
Compare two paired groups	Paired *t* test	Wilcoxon test	McNemar's test
Compare three or more unmatched groups	One-way ANOVA	Kruskal-Wallis test	Chi-square test
Compare three or more matched groups	Repeated-measures ANOVA	Friedman test	Cochrane Q
Quantify association between two variables	Pearson correlation	Spearman correlation	Contingency coefficients
Predict value from another measured variable	Simple linear regression or nonlinear regression	Nonparametric regression	Simple logistic regression
Predict value from several measured or binomial variables	Multiple linear regression or multiple nonlinear regression		Multiple logistic regression

Exercise 7

Aim of the study is to see the effect of prolonged and high dose of corticosteroid on severity of wheezing after the infection of RSV (respiratory syncytial virus).

First question: What is the aim?

Here, the aim is "compare two unpaired groups". One group is drug group and another is placebo group.

Second question: What type of data it is?

The number of days of wheezing is nominal data.

Third question: Whether the data follow the normal distribution?

Nominal data do not follow the normal distribution.

So, on the basis of table, the most appropriate test in this condition will be "Fisher's test". Here, sample size is big so even Chi-square could have been used.

	Type of data		
Goal	Ratio and interval data which follows normal distribution	Ratio and interval data which does not follow normal distribution and ordinal data (rank and scores)	Nominal data
Describe one group	Mean, standard deviation	Median, interquartile range	Proportion
Compare one group to a hypothetical value	One-sample *t* test	Wilcoxon test	Chi-square or binomial test
Compare two unpaired groups	Unpaired *t* test	Mann-Whitney test	Fisher's test (Chi-square for large samples)

(*Contd.*)

(*Contd.*)

	Type of data		
Compare two paired groups	Paired *t* test	Wilcoxon test	McNemar's test
Compare three or more unmatched groups	One-way ANOVA	Kruskal-Wallis test	Chi-square test
Compare three or more matched groups	Repeated-measures ANOVA	Friedman test	Cochrane Q
Quantify association between two variables	Pearson correlation	Spearman correlation	Contingency coefficients
Predict value from another measured variable	Simple linear regression or nonlinear regression	Nonparametric regression	Simple logistic regression
Predict value from several measured or binomial variables	Multiple linear regression or multiple nonlinear regression		Multiple logistic regression

Exercise 8

In the case of survival time we should know the goal so appropriate test can be selected.

Question: What is the aim?

Aim is to "compare two unpaired group".

For this aim "log-rank test or Mantel-Haenszel test" will be appropriate. Two Kaplan Meier curve can be compared by these tests.

Goal	Test
Describe one group	Kaplan Meier survival curve
Compare one group to a hypothetical value	
Compare two unpaired groups	Log-rank test or Mantel-Haenszel
Compare two paired groups	Conditional proportional hazards regression
Compare three or more unmatched groups	Cox proportional hazard regression
Compare three or more matched groups	Conditional proportional hazards regression
Quantify association between two variables	
Predict value from another measured variable	Cox proportional hazard regression
Predict value from several measured or binomial variables	Cox proportional hazard regression

Exercise 9

In this study researcher's interest is in knowing the effect of extract of Tinospora cordifolia on various blood parameters in the patients of HIV/AIDS. Separate tests need to be used for each parameter. Here, all parameters are of ratio data so same test will be used for each parameters.

First question: What is the aim?

Here, the aim is "compare two unpaired groups". One group is herb group and another is placebo group.

Second question: What type of data it is?

All blood parameters are ratio data.

Third question: Whether the data follow the normal distribution?

Data do not follow the normal distribution.

So, on the basis of table, the most appropriate test in this condition will be "Mann-Whitney test".

	Type of data		
Goal	Ratio and interval data which follows normal distribution	Ratio and interval data which does not follow normal distribution and ordinal data (rank and scores)	Nominal data
Describe one group	Mean, SD	Median, interquartile range	Proportion
Compare one group to a hypothetical value	One-sample *t* test	Wilcoxon test	Chi-square or binomial test
Compare two unpaired groups	Unpaired *t* test	Mann-Whitney test	Fisher's test (Chi-square for large samples)
Compare two paired groups	Paired *t* test	Wilcoxon test	McNemar's test
Compare three or more unmatched groups	One-way ANOVA	Kruskal-Wallis test	Chi-square test
Compare three or more matched groups	Repeated-measures ANOVA	Friedman test	Cochrane Q

(Contd.)

(*Contd.*)

	Type of data		
Quantify association between two variables	Pearson correlation	Spearman correlation	Contingency coefficients
Predict value from another measured variable	Simple linear regression or nonlinear regression	Nonparametric regression	Simple logistic regression
Predict value from several measured or binomial variables	Multiple linear regression or multiple nonlinear regression		Multiple logistic regression

Index